OSCEs in
Obstetrics and Gynaecology
for MRCOG-3

OSCEs in
Obstetrics and Gynaecology
for MRCOG-3

Richa Saxena MBBS MD (OB-GYN)
PG Diploma in Clinical Research
Obstetrician and Gynaecologist
New Delhi, India

JAYPEE *The Health Sciences Publisher*

New Delhi | London | Panama

Jaypee Brothers Medical Publishers (P) Ltd

Headquarters

Jaypee Brothers Medical Publishers (P) Ltd
4838/24, Ansari Road, Daryaganj
New Delhi 110 002, India
Phone: +91-11-43574357
Fax: +91-11-43574314
Email: jaypee@jaypeebrothers.com

Overseas Offices

J.P. Medical Ltd
83 Victoria Street, London
SW1H 0HW (UK)
Phone: +44-20 317 08910
Fax: +44 (0)20 3008 6180
Email: info@jpmedpub.com

Jaypee Brothers Medical Publishers (P) Ltd
17/1-B Babar Road, Block-B, Shyamoli
Mohammadpur, Dhaka-1207
Bangladesh
Mobile: +08801912003485
Email: jaypeedhaka@gmail.com

Jaypee-Highlights Medical Publishers Inc
City of Knowledge, Bld. 235, 2nd floor, Clayton
Panama City, Panama
Phone: +1 507-301-0496
Fax: +1 507-301-0499
Email: cservice@jphmedical.com

Jaypee Brothers Medical Publishers (P) Ltd
Bhotahity, Kathmandu, Nepal
Phone: +977-9741283608
Email: Kathmandu@jaypeebrothers.com

Website: www.jaypeebrothers.com
Website: www.jaypeedigital.com

OSCEs in Obstetrics and Gynaecology for MRCOG-3

First Edition: 2018

ISBN 978-93-5270-381-4

Printed at Sanat Printers

Dedicated to...

My mother Mrs Bharati Saxena for always being there.....
My mother was the most beautiful woman I ever saw. All I am
I owe to my mother. I attribute all my success in life to the moral,
intellectual and physical education, I received from her."

—**George Washington**

Preface

A good physician treats the disease; the great physician treats the patient who has the disease.

—William Osler

As the saying goes, treatment of a patient encompasses much more than the treatment of the disease. The MRCOG Part 3 examination is exactly based on this principle and tests doctors' skills for treating patients, their way of communicating with them, exhibiting empathy towards them, dealing with them, applying their clinical knowledge and then treating them. Having written books for MRCOG Part 1 and Part 2 examinations, I felt there was a requirement for books on the clinical examination or OSCEs for the part 3 examination. Initially, the OSCE examination was a component of the MRCOG Part 2 examination. However, since September 2016 there has been a change in the examination pattern. Now, the part 2 examination constitutes only of the written component. The clinical skills are tested as another standalone examination or the MRCOG Part 3 examination. Though this examination is considered to be difficult, if the candidates acquire certain skills they are likely to sail through the examination with flying colours. This book has been written with precisely this intention in mind. The book would provide an orientation to the readers to successfully attempt the OSCE stations. There are nearly 40 OSCE scenarios in the book. Each station presents the likely variations that can be encountered during the examination. Furthermore, each station discusses the issues related to clinical management as well as clinical governance. A separate chapter on clinical governance has also been provided. The structure of healthcare system (National Health Services) in the UK and the role of midwives in the care of pregnant women have also been discussed in details, especially for the overseas candidates.

The text aptly offers all the required information a specialist registrar or senior house officer requires during his/her training period and while preparing for the MRCOG examination. In fact, this book would also assist all the applicants, especially overseas, preparing for MRCOG examination (Parts 2 and 3).

I believe that writing a book involves a continuous learning process. Though extreme care has been taken to maintain the accuracy while writing this book, constructive criticism would be greatly appreciated. Please e-mail me your comments at the e-mail address: richa@drrichasaxena.com. Also, please feel free to visit my website www.drrichasaxena.com for obtaining relevant information of various other books written by me and to make use of the free online resources available for the doctors attempting the

MRCOG examination. To help the doctors attempt and clear the various parts of the MRCOG examination, Jaypee Brothers Medical Publishers has also launched an e-learning platform, cracking MRCOG (mentored by me). If interested in knowing more about this platform, kindly visit the website www.crackingmrcog.com.

Richa Saxena MBBS MD
richa@drrichasaxena.com
www.drrichasaxena.com

Acknowledgment

Writing a book is a colossal task. It can never be completed without divine intervention and approval. Therefore, I have decided to start this acknowledgment with a small prayer of thanks to the Almighty, which I was taught in my childhood.

"Father, lead me day by day, ever in thy own sweet way. Teach me to be pure and good and tell me what I ought to do."

—Amen

Simultaneously, I would like to extend my thanks and appreciation to all the related authors and publishers whose references have been used in this book. Book creation is teamwork and I acknowledge the way the entire staff of M/s Jaypee Brothers Medical Publishers (P) Ltd., New Delhi, India, worked hard on this manuscript to give it a final shape. I would especially like to thank Mr Jitendar P Vij (Group Chairman), Mr Ankit Vij (Group President), Mr Yogeshwar Pal (medical editor), Mr Sunil Rawat (typesetter), Mr Gopal Singh (artist), and Ms Seema Dogra (cover designer) for publishing and giving a final shape to this book.

Richa Saxena MBBS MD
richa@drrichasaxena.com
www.drrichasaxena.com

Contents

Abbreviations

MRCOG: Member of the Royal College of Obstetricians and Gynaecologists
RCOG: Royal College of Obstetricians and Gynaecologists
CCT: Certificate of Completion of Training
ST: Specialty Training
FY: Foundation Training
OSCE: Objective Structured Clinical Examination
EPALS: The European Paediatric Advanced Life Support
NICE: National Institute for Health and Care Excellence
NHS: National Health Service
GMC: General Medical Council
TOG: The Obstetrician & Gynaecologist
CPD: Continuing Professional Development
PIH: Pregnancy-induced Hypertension
IUGR: Intrauterine Growth Restriction
VBAC: Vaginal Birth After Caesarean
GP: General Practitioner
PALS: Patient Advice and Liaison Services
APGAR: Appearance, Pulse, Grimace, Activity, Respiration
CCG: Clinical Commissioning Group
MCV: Mean Corpuscular Volume
GTT: Glucose Tolerance Test
DIC: Disseminated Intravascular Coagulation
FFP: Fresh Frozen Plasma
CVP: Central Venous Pressure
CNST: Clinical Negligence Scheme for Trusts
NPSA: National Patient Safety Agency
CQC: Care Quality Commission
NICU: Neonatal Intensive Care Unit
A&E: Accident and Emergency
HIE: Hypoxic Ischaemic Encephalopathy
CMACE: Centre for Maternal and Child Enquiries
OSAT: Objective Structured Assessment of Technical Skills
ALSO: Advanced Life Support in Obstetrics
UTI: Urinary Tract Infection
VTE: Venous Thromboembolism
DVT: Deep Vein Thrombosis
IVU: Intravenous Urography
FBC: Full Blood Count
IV: Intravenous
VE: Vaginal Examination
CTG: Cardiotocography

hCG: Human Chorionic Gonadotropin
JW: Jehovah's Witness
HIV: Human Immunodeficiency Virus
GUM: Genitourinary Medicine
IUI: Intrauterine Insemination
IVF: In Vitro Fertilisation
HVS: High Vaginal Swab
LMP: Last Menstrual Period
EDD: Expected Date of Delivery
MSU: Midstream Urine
VDRL: Venereal Disease Research Laboratory
FSH: Follicle-stimulating Hormone
LH: Luteinising Hormone
CIN: Cervical Intraepithelial Neoplasia
MLU: Midwifery-led Unit
FBS: Foetal Blood Sample
IM: Intramuscular
FHR: Foetal Heart Rate
BP: Blood Pressure
PCOS: Polycystic Ovarian Syndrome
EPU: Early Pregnancy Unit

1

Training in Obstetrics and Gynaecology in the UK

INTRODUCTION

The Royal College of Obstetricians and Gynaecologists (RCOG) has developed a curriculum for specialty training in obstetrics and gynaecology in the UK.[1] The main aim of this specialty training curriculum for obstetrics and gynaecology is competency instead of considering variable steps or the amount of time spent on the training. As a result, it may take longer time for some trainees to achieve all competencies and their certificate of completion of training (CCT) as compared to others. Candidates who are starting at specialty training year 1 (ST1) level can expect to take 7 years for completing their training, subject to satisfactory assessment of progress. The number of posts available at ST1 to ST3 (specialty training year 3) level varies each year across the UK.

CAREER PATHWAY IN OBSTETRICS AND GYNAECOLOGY

If the aspirants are thinking to pursue a career in obstetrics and gynaecology following their graduation in medicine, they are advised to gain as much experience as possible before applying for the specialty training. Before applying for specialty training in obstetrics and gynaecology, candidates must ensure that they develop appropriate skills required to be a good obstetrician and gynaecologist. Some examples of these skills are as follows: clinical problem solving, good communication skills, decision making, teamwork, empathy, sensitivity, manual dexterity, working under pressure, etc.[2] Day-to-day management and quality assurance of training are provided by the postgraduate dean during the period of specialty training. Alternatively, the training programme director supervises the training programme at the local level.

When the candidate enters specialty training programme in obstetrics and gynaecology, they would be provided with an ePortfolio by the RCOG.[3] This portfolio shall act as a log for the attainment of competencies in the curriculum.

It also records their inductions and appraisals as well as workplace-based assessment. The RCOG and the concerned deanery shall keep in touch with the candidate via the ePortfolio.

Throughout the candidate's training period, the College shall set out the criteria and content for training. They will also provide guidance regarding the educational support material and training courses. Figure 1.1 represents the training programme in obstetrics and gynaecology in the UK and this training programme is also described next in details.

TRAINING PROGRAMME IN OBSTETRICS AND GYNAECOLOGY

The candidates who are considering their career in obstetrics and gynaecology can apply for specialty training, which is a run-through scheme, following the completion of their foundation training (FY1 and FY2). Aspirants apply for training at ST1 level. Advancement to ST2 level, and then to ST3 and beyond (till the ST7 level) occurs; only if candidates are successful at subsequent levels. When the applicant has accomplished all the requirements of the programme, they will be awarded a Certificate of Completion of Training and registered in the specialist register of the General Medical Council.[1] They can then practice at the consultant level in the UK.

Application process for specialty training in obstetrics and gynaecology is a competitive process initiated via the Health Education North West website (https://www.nwpgmd.nhs.uk/OG_Recruitment).[4] The responsibility for national recruitment to obstetrics and gynaecology at ST1 level has been formally transferred by the Health Education England from the Royal College of Obstetricians and Gynaecologists to Health Education North West with effect from the August 2017 intake. In 2016, the competition ratio of clinical trainee to specialty trainee (CT1:ST1) in Obstetrics and Gynaecology was 2.03.[5]

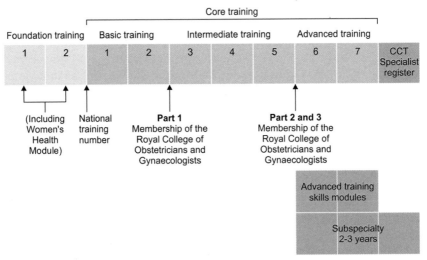

Fig. 1.1: Career pathway for obstetrics and gynaecology.[1]
(CCT: certificate of completion of training)

There were 2,133 consultants and 2,481 medical registrars in England in the year 2016 in the specialty of obstetrics and gynaecology.[6]

Foundation Training (FY1 and FY2)

A rotation in obstetrics and gynaecology is involved in many posts for foundation year 2 and a few posts for foundation year 1. For the candidates who have just completed their medical graduation and are interested in further pursuing their career in the field of obstetrics and gynaecology, it is a wise decision to spend some time doing an audit, publishing a case report, or conducting teaching sessions in the specialty of obstetrics and gynaecology. Presently, MRCOG part 1 of the examination can be attempted as soon as you have gained your medical degree. Successfully clearing the Membership of the Royal College of Obstetricians and Gynaecologists (MRCOG) Part 1 examination during the foundation training is likely to help you gain an edge over the other candidates while applying for the ST1 post in obstetrics and gynaecology.

During the foundation programme, the candidates who are wishing to pursue their specialty training in the field of obstetrics and gynaecology are expected to complete the Women's Health Module available on the RCOG website. Prior to the submission of an application for specialty training, it is essential for the candidate in the previous 1 year to undertake a formal hands-on training on basic life support. This may be undertaken in a hospital posting or on a recognised course. Other desirable courses which can be attempted by the candidates prior to the application for ST1 post include various courses such as:

- *The basic practical skills in obstetrics and gynaecology course*: The content of this course is designed to complement the RCOG Training Portfolio Logbook and is linked to OSATs or Objective Structured Assessment of Technical skills.
- *The Advanced Life Support in Obstetrics (ALSO) course*: This is an evidence-based, interprofessional, and multidisciplinary training programme. This training programme equips the entire maternity team to effectively manage various obstetric emergencies.
- *The European Paediatric Advanced Life Support (EPALS) course*: It is a collaborative course between the European Resuscitation Council and the Resuscitation Council (UK). The aim of EPALS is to train the doctors and nurses in the efficient and prompt management of the children showing early signs of respiratory or circulatory failure.

Core Training

Years 1 and 2 (ST1 and ST2): Basic Specialty Training

Aspirants are likely to gain knowledge and skills in several areas of obstetrics and gynaecology at ST1 and ST2 level, while working together with other trainees at the similar level as well as those at advanced levels. Though the candidate is likely to work with several consultants across a range of specialties, there would be one consultant who would act as their educational supervisor.

After satisfactory completion of the required assessments, the candidate is likely to progress to ST2. Within a minimum span of 2 years at the level of ST1-2, the candidate is likely to achieve all the required competencies.

The candidate is expected to see the patients in antenatal and gynaecology clinics during the basic specialty training. An opportunity to do caesarean sections and conduct instrumental deliveries in the delivery suite will also be provided to them. There are many other competencies required for the candidate at ST1 and ST2 level besides conducting uncomplicated elective caesarean sections and non-rotational instrumental deliveries and those include opening and closing the abdomen during various surgeries, perineal repair, and uncomplicated surgical uterine evacuation.[7] The training achievements of all individuals will be recorded in their training logbook and ePortfolio.[3]

With the advancement of candidate's training, they will start to possess the various competencies in their logbook signed off. After the candidates attain set competencies and are successful in their annual review of competence progression, they are able to reach to the next level of their specialty training.

Progression from ST2 to ST3 Level

One of the important assessment steps of progression from ST2 to ST3 level (i.e. from basic to intermediate training) for a candidate is to pass the first part of the RCOG membership examination (Part 1 MRCOG). They should have completed the RCOG basic practical skills in obstetrics and gynaecology course, and should have attained the relevant competencies for independent practice as highlighted in the trainee logbook. This includes modules in basic clinical and surgical skills, teaching appraisal and assessment, ethical and legal issues, and maternal medicine. At this stage, the candidate is likely to take increased clinical responsibility and progresses from first on call to second on call. At this level, the candidates become competent to handle the delivery suite independently. At the same time, they must be aware of their limitations and should know when to seek senior assistance.

Years 3–5 (ST3–ST5): Intermediate Training

Once the candidates have progressed to ST3 level, they will have to spend the next 3 years obtaining further experience in all areas in the specialty of obstetrics and gynaecology. By the time, the candidates reach ST4 to ST5 level, they have become capable to carry out almost all the obstetric and gynaecological procedures with indirect supervision (with a consultant available nearby). By the time candidates reach ST5 level, they have acquired a broad base of knowledge and expertise on which to develop advanced skills and make future career plans. During this time, trainees get the opportunity to follow their subspecialty interests. They get a chance to work closely with a consultant in a specific subspecialty. Satisfactory completion of ST5 marks the completion of intermediate training.

To progress through training during ST3 to ST5 levels, the candidates need to achieve set competencies as mentioned in their ePortfolios and logbooks.

They also need to have regular assessments. In order to progress towards advanced training (ST6 level) following the completion of intermediate training, the candidate needs to complete all the intermediate competencies and pass the second part of the membership examination (Part 2 and Part 3 MRCOG examination). Once the candidate has completed all intermediate requirements, they move to ST6 level. Here they have the option to complete advanced training skills modules (ATSMs) or do subspecialty training.

Years 6 and 7 (ST6 and ST7): Advanced Training

During ST6 and ST7 level, the candidates continue to expand and improve their general skills in obstetrics and gynaecology. Besides consolidating the clinical skills they have already learned during specialty training, they are likely to expand their knowledge in topics such as medical management and clinical governance. This would ensure that they are properly prepared for the non-clinical aspects of working as a consultant in the National Health Service (NHS).

During this period, the candidates also get a chance to gain more knowledge and experience in their area of special interest. They have the option to do ATSM or the subspecialty training.[8] Following these two final 2 years of training, the candidate can apply for their final qualification, the Certificate of Completion of Training.

Advanced training skills modules: The candidate can choose from 20 ATSMs, based on the skills suitable for future career progress as a consultant. Some of the advanced training modules include, maternal medicine, oncology, forensic gynaecology, vulval disease, medical education, and menopause.[9]

Subspecialty training: Subspecialists are obstetricians and gynaecologists who are recognized to have subspecialty expertise in their field. They have undertaken appropriate additional higher training beyond that which can be achieved in normal advanced training. There are four subspecialties in obstetrics and gynaecology: gynaecological oncology, maternal and foetal medicine, reproductive medicine, urogynaecology and sexual and reproductive healthcare. The training programme is set out by the relevant subspecialty. The candidate would, however, continue to undertake on call work in general obstetrics and gynaecology during their subspecialty training. The subspecialty training lasts for 3 years: 2 years of clinical training and 1 year of research. If the candidate has already published appropriate publications, it may count towards the research component.

CERTIFICATION OF TRAINING AND SPECIALIST REGISTRATION

For the candidates to be able to practice as a consultant in the NHS, they need to be entered on the Specialist Register. On successful completion of their advanced training, they would be conferred certificate of completion of training. The RCOG would then recommend them to the General Medical Council for inclusion on the Specialist Register. This would enable the candidate to independently practice as a consultant in obstetrics and gynaecology in the UK.

NATIONAL HEALTH SERVICES

While attempting the MRCOG Part 2 or 3 examination, it is especially important for the overseas candidates to be familiar with the working of healthcare system in the UK. NHS or the National Health Service is a publicly funded national healthcare system for England. The four national health services in the United Kingdom include NHS (England), NHS (Scotland), NHS (Northern Ireland), and NHS (Wales).[10] It is the largest and oldest single-payer healthcare system in the world and covers all healthcare services including the antenatal care, screenings, maternity services, long-term healthcare, and end of life care. Three core principles of NHS are as follows:

1. Based on clinical needs and not on the ability to pay
2. Meeting the requirements of everyone
3. Free at the point of delivery.

Funding for NHS directly comes from taxation. Various levels of healthcare in the NHS include primary level, secondary level, and tertiary level. As per data of March 2017, there are 233 NHS providers of secondary and tertiary care. Of these 233 NHS providers, there are 152 foundation trusts and 81 aspirant trusts.[11] Additional non-NHS organisations also provide secondary and tertiary care services.

Primary Level Healthcare

Primary care acts as the first point of contact for someone and covers everyday health services. It can be regarded as the 'gateway' to receiving more specialist care. It is usually delivered by primary care trusts such as GPs (general practitioners), dentists or opticians. NHS provides funds to the GP surgeries that are responsible for delivering primary care to the patients. There is a clinic called GP surgery in every community, which covers the population in their catchment area. People living in that area can get themselves registered with that GP surgery. The medical records of a person are usually held by the GP. The GP also knows the patient's complete medical history. Patients usually cannot refer themselves to a specialist except in two conditions:

1. Referral to A&E
2. Referral to sexual health clinics or genitourinary medicine (GUM clinics).

All the preliminary work-up of the patients before referring them to the secondary care (hospitals) is usually done at the GP surgery. When the patient is referred to secondary or tertiary care, the GP surgery pays the hospital for that visit. Therefore, hospitals earn money through these referrals. No payment is done for any further follow-up. As a result, the patients are usually followed up in the GP surgeries based on the recommendations made by the specialists. The specialist may call the patient for further follow-up based on their discretion depending upon the patient's clinical condition.

Secondary Level Healthcare

Secondary level healthcare includes hospital-based as well as community-based care. It can either be planned (elective) care such as a cataract operation, or urgent and emergency care such as treatment for a fracture. Hospital-based care is usually provided by the specialists. A patient is referred to a secondary care professional from primary care. A specialist in secondary or tertiary care will see only those patients who have a referral letter from GP, which outlines the patient's background, the treatments initiated so far, and the patient's response to treatment. Once the specialists have seen the patient, they would write back to the GP their recommendations and observations. Based on the results of the observations or investigations, the specialist may decide to call the patient back to the hospital or refer them back to the GP for further follow-up. In either case, a letter is issued to the GP updating regarding what was done. For example, if the specialist discovers a microbial growth on high vaginal swab (HVS), they can refer the patient back to the GP who would then prescribe appropriate antibiotics to the patient. On the other hand, if the investigation reveals CIN, the patient would be referred to the hospital's colposcopy clinic.

Tertiary Level Healthcare

Tertiary level of healthcare is known as specialized consultative healthcare. This type of healthcare service is usually for inpatients and on referral from primary and secondary healthcare for advanced medical investigation and treatment.

ANTENATAL CARE (MIDWIFERY SYSTEM) IN THE UK

Midwifery system prevails in UK for the care of pregnant women. Midwives act as lead professionals for providing maternity care to all healthy pregnant women. They deliver all aspects of pregnant woman's physical, psychological, and social care. They also act as the first point of contact for the women who want to access maternity services. In case of complicated pregnancies, midwives act as the prime co-ordinators of care within the multidisciplinary team, where they closely work with the obstetricians, GP, specialist services, social services, breast feeding services, etc.

Midwives can conduct a normal vaginal delivery, suture episiotomies, and repair first and second degree tears. In the maternity triage and antenatal day care assessment, midwives can check a patient's presentation and treat the patient on their own unless they encounter a problem and feel the requirement to involve a doctor. In the NHS, following grades of midwives are available: student midwives, middle grade midwives, senior midwives, and specialist midwives. In the UK, midwives can work in the following sectors as discussed next.

Community Level

Community level midwives provide home visits to the patients, antenatal care, postnatal assessments, assessment of the patient's social support needs, etc.

Hospital Level

- *Hospital obstetric units*: Each pregnant patient gets one-to-one midwifery care in the hospital's labour room. The doctors are only involved in the patient's care if the midwives feel requirement for the same.

- *Midwife led unit (MLU)*: These are separate birth centres other than the labour room where the midwives conduct delivery themselves without using any medical intervention. These units are usually next to the main hospital's maternity unit. Facilities for water birth are also here. In case any complication is anticipated during labour, the midwife would advise the patient to change her plan and deliver in the obstetric unit.

In the NHS, the obstetricians or doctors are involved in antenatal care or delivery of patients only when the midwife encounters a complication or feel the requirement for their involvement.

SUMMARY

Obstetrics and gynaecology is a unique specialty which is a combination of both medicine and surgery. This specialty is not only concerned with the care of pregnant woman and her unborn child, but also the management of diseases specific to women. A career in obstetrics and gynaecology is likely to be both thrilling and rewarding due to the broad range of subspecialties it offers. It presents countless opportunities, enabling the budding obstetrician and gynaecologist to practise high-quality medicine in an atmosphere of multidisciplinary team. A career in obstetrics and gynaecology in the UK warrants an understanding regarding the working of NHS as well as the role of midwives in imparting care to the pregnant women.

REFERENCES

1. Royal College of Obstetricians and gynaecologists. (2017). About speciality training in obstetrics and gynaecology. [online] Available from https://www.rcog.org.uk/en/careers-training/about-specialty-training-in-og/ [Accessed July 2017].
2. Health Careers. (2017). Obstetrics and gynaecology. [online] Available from https://www.healthcareers.nhs.uk/explore-roles/obstetrics-and-gynaecology [Accessed July 2017].
3. ePortfolio. NHS ePortfolio. [online] Available from https://www.nhseportfolios.org [Accessed July 2017].
4. Health Education England North West. (2016). Obstetrics & Gynaecology Recruitment. [online] Available from https://www.nwpgmd.nhs.uk/OG_Recruitment [Accessed July 2017].
5. NHS specialty training. (2016). 2016 – CT1/ST1 Competition Ratios. [online] Available from https://specialtytraining.hee.nhs.uk/Portals/1/Competition%20Ratios%202016%20ST1_1.pdf [Accessed July 2017].
6. NHS digital. (2017). NHS Workforce Statistics - December 2016, Provisional statistics. [online] Available from http://content.digital.nhs.uk/home [Accessed July 2017].
7. Oxford deanery. (2017). Obstetrics and Gynaecology - ST1 - person specification -2017. [online] Available from http://www.oxforddeanery.nhs.uk/pdf/OG-PS-ST1-1232017-1.pdf [Accessed July 2017].
8. Rimmer A. (2017). Postgraduate training will be more flexible under new standards, says GMC. [online] Available from http://careers.bmj.com/careers/advice/Postgraduate_training_will_be_more_flexible_under_new_standards%2C_says_GMC [Accessed July 2017].

9. Abdelrahman A, McNeill S. (2012). A career in obstetrics and gynaecology. BMJ Careers. [online] Available from http://careers.bmj.com/careers/advice/view-article.html?id=20008722 [Accessed July 2017].

10. NHS choices. (2016). About the National Health Service. [online] Available from https://www.nhs.uk/NHSEngland/thenhs/about/Pages/overview.aspx [Accessed December 2017].

11. NHS confederation. (2017). NHS statistics, facts and figures. [online] Available from http://www.nhsconfed.org/resources/key-statistics-on-the-nhs [Accessed December 2017].

2

Basics of the MRCOG Part 3 Examination

INTRODUCTION

The Part 2 and the Part 3 MRCOG examinations aim at evaluating the skills that are expected of an ST5 (specialist trainee 5), who has completed core and intermediate training, in the clinical practice of obstetrics and gynaecology as practiced in the National Health Service (NHS). To do well in the examination, the candidates just need to perform all their clinical activities as they would have normally done in the clinic, ward, theatre or labour ward as an ST5 trainee. The MRCOG is a licensing examination and the Royal College of Obstetricians and Gynaecologists (RCOG) needs to be sure that the candidate is competent enough to independently practice at a consultant level, following the completion of their training.

It is a criterion-referenced and not a norm-referenced examination. In a criterion-referenced examination, the minimum standard acceptable for passing the examination has already been decided before the test. If you are able to reach that particular standard, you pass. Else, if you get marks below that standard, you fail. As a result, the standard required to pass the MRCOG Part 3 examination remains consistent between examinations irrespective of the relative difficulty of a particular examination.

On the other hand, in a norm-referenced examination, the candidate's performance is evaluated in comparison with the performance of other candidates. Therefore, you may be disadvantaged, if the other candidates attempting the examination are more experienced. Similarly, you may be advantaged, if the other candidates attempting the examination are less experienced.

FORMAT OF MRCOG PART 3 EXAMINATION

Currently, the Part 3 MRCOG examination comprises of 14 tasks, each relating to one of the 14 modules to be assessed by the curriculum of MRCOG

Part 3 examination.[1] Each task is 12 minutes in length. This is inclusive of 2 minutes of initial reading time. At the beginning of each task, candidates are given 2 minutes outside the booth to read the background information and instructions for the task. When the 2 minutes of reading time is over, the buzzer will sound and candidates will enter the booth. They must then start attempting the task. The examiner and the role-player would be inside the booth. For some stations, there may be no role-player, just the examiner. The information exhibited outside the booth will also be replicated inside the booth, usually attached to the desk. Once 10 minutes are over, the buzzer would sound again. This is an indicator for the candidate that the particular station is over and they need to move onto the next station. The sound of the buzzer is also an indicator for the examiner to mark the candidate. This process goes on until the candidate has encountered all the 14 stations. As a result, the duration of examination is approximately 3 hours.

OBJECTIVE STRUCTURED CLINICAL EXAMINATION (OSCE)

To avoid many of the disadvantages of the traditional clinical examination, the model of OSCE has been introduced.[2] In this type of examination pattern, the students rotate around a series of structured stations. The candidates may be required to carry out different tasks at various stations; for example, at one station the candidate may be required to break bad news to the patient; at the second station, they may be required to take a history; at the third one to interpret the provided laboratory investigations in the light of a patient's problem, and so on. At each of these stations, the candidate is required to perform a defined set of tasks. The examiner may also ask the candidate a few questions. The candidate needs to perform the required tasks and provide the answers to the questions asked by the examiner. The examiner marks the candidate at the end of each station using a pre-defined marksheet. Since the marking is carried out in real time, no marks are forgotten, thereby eliminating the possibility of recall bias. Also, this type of examination pattern reduces the possibility for the candidate to go back and check their omissions, which they can do in case of written examination. As a result, the structured clinical examination helps in easily controlling the variables and complexity of the examination, clearly defining its aims and carrying out an accurate assessment of the student's knowledge.

There can be two types of OSCE stations in the Part 3 MRCOG examination: simulated patient or colleague tasks and structured discussion tasks.

Simulated Patient or Colleague Tasks

These are the tasks where the candidate interacts with an actor (role-player). The examiner would be present in such stations in order to assess the candidate. However, they would neither interact with the role-player nor the candidate. The candidate must also not interact with the examiner on these stations. The simulated patient tasks are similar to the cases encountered by ST5 in the NHS wards and clinics.

Role-Players

In the simulated patient or colleague task, the candidates interact with actors who have been trained and instructed about the role they are supposed to play. The actors are provided with all the significant details concerning the case. They are also given some scripted questions to prompt the candidate in case it is required. They have been instructed to display emotions appropriate to the scenario; for example, they may get angry, anxious, or upset depending on the situation. However, they would not demonstrate extreme of emotions such as shouting or swearing. Also, they will not leave the station during the 10 minutes of the examination time. These actors are proficient at improvisation and they would provide clues to the candidates in case they are going in the wrong direction. So, it is important for the candidate to carefully observe the role-player's facial expressions during the task.

The role-player in front of the candidate may not have similar physical and demographic characteristics as the one described in the stated clinical scenario. However, it is important for the candidate to appreciate this aspect. For example, if the role-player does not have raised body mass index (BMI), but the clinical scenario described for a particular OSCE station describes the patient to be having a raised BMI, then the candidate must consider that the BMI of the role-player is raised in the context of that particular OSCE station. Similarly, the candidate may encounter a young role-player playing the character of a woman in her late 50s. Again, the candidate must consider her age as described in the clinical scenario and not on the basis of her physical appearance. Therefore, it is extremely important for the candidate to carefully read the patient's background details provided in the clinical scenario of that particular OSCE station and conduct the task according to the written instructions. The candidates must not go by the apparent physical characteristics of the actor. In case the candidate cannot recall the details they had read before entering the examination booth, they must remember that the similar details of the clinical scenario shall also be affixed to their table inside the examination booth. So they need not panic!

The role-players are given the authority to award up to 2 marks to the candidate depending on their confidence on the doctor and whether they would be prepared to see that doctor (candidate) again in future.

Prior to the examination, there is a detailed training session for the role-players or simulated patients to help ensure that they have fully understood the role they are supposed to play as defined in their instructions. This drill also helps in ensuring that they perform their tasks in standard manner in each circuit in the examination centre so that all the candidates are evaluated in a similar manner.

Role of Examiner

In a simulated patient (or colleague) task, the examiner would be present in the examination booth. However, they will not interact with the candidate or the role-player. They will be observing the candidate with a neutral facial expression and taking notes. They would be awarding marks to the candidate during each task. The candidate must remember not to interact with them or explain them anything.

Examiners

Candidates can be evaluated by two types of examiners: the clinical examiners and the lay examiners. In at least four of the simulated patient tasks in any single examination there may be both a clinical examiner and a lay examiner.

Clinical Examiners

All the clinical examiners for MRCOG Part 3 examination are fellows or members of the RCOG and in current clinical practice. All these examiners have been formally trained in conducting the examination, evaluating the candidate's clinical skills, and awarding them marks. Prior to each examination, there is a comprehensive meeting where the examiners are given instructions about a particular task. There is a detailed review of the examination scenario, examination instructions, and the marking scheme. This detailed training session ensures that assessment of each candidate is carried out against the same criteria and level of skills, thereby ensuring fairness in marking each candidate. This training also helps in ensuring that the examiner well understands the level of knowledge, skills and competencies, which a ST5 trainee must possess, and the appropriate professional attitudes and behaviours which they must exhibit in order to pass the MRCOG examination. The standard required for the candidate to pass in each of the tasks and domains is decided during the examiner's briefing session, well before the start of the examination.

Lay Examiners

The involvement of lay examiners in the assessment of doctors is based on the contemporary approach to obstetrics and gynaecology in which patients are anticipated to be partners in their own care and expected to be involved in shared decision-making regarding the management of their disease. Persons chosen to act as lay examiners are generally recruited from the general public. They do not have any clinical training or background in order to ensure that they accurately represent the vast majority of patients that obstetricians and gynaecologists encounter on a daily basis. All lay examiners, however, undergo an initial recruitment and selection process as well as an arduous training programme to help understand their role within the Part 3 MRCOG examination.

The task of lay examiners is to mark the communication skills of the candidates while they are interacting with the role-players (patients) and/or their families. Lay examiners also undergo a training sessions for the tasks they will be examining, along with the clinical examiners and actors. Similar to the clinical examiners, the lay examiners award marks in real time during the task and in the 2 minutes at the end of each task after the candidate has left the examination booth.

Structured Discussion Tasks

In the structured discussion tasks, the candidate directly interacts with the examiner. The role-player is not present on these stations. In these cases, the examiner will have detailed instructions about the task. They would also have a list of prompt questions to ensure that the candidate moves in the right direction. The examiner may provide further information (e.g. results of investigations or more clinical details) to the candidate as the scenario evolves and then ask further questions. They may also ask the candidate to explain or further expand on an answer. These tasks may be similar to having case-based discussion with the consultant either on the ward round or while phoning them out of hours. These tasks could also be simulating a handover been given to a colleague or tasks related to the principles of clinical governance. These kind of situations may arise every working day, where information is exchanged and the consultant clarifies details or asks for further information where required.

The examiner's aim is not to fail the candidate, but to ensure that all candidates having the basic knowledge, skills, attitudes, and competencies are able to pass the MRCOG examination. All examiners are trained to ensure that candidates are given adequate opportunity to demonstrate their skills. If the examiner feels that the candidate is not moving on the right track, they may ask them prompt questions to ensure that they are moving in the right direction. This helps in confirming that the candidate is able to cover all aspects of a particular clinical scenario in the time available. This way the candidates get the best chance to demonstrate all their skills.

Linked Tasks

In the Part 3 MRCOG examination, some of the OSCE tasks may be linked to each other. One station may represent a scenario representing a particular module, which may be linked to another station representing another module. For example, there could be a task related to antenatal management (Module 4) in a patient with placenta praevia. This station may evolve into a scenario related to a difficult caesarean delivery. This station would be then related to another module, i.e. Module 7 (Management of Delivery) in this case. This OSCE station is likely to deal with different issues in comparison to the previous station. Therefore, it is important for the candidate to know that although clinical scenarios in two separate OSCE stations may be linked, each of the tasks would be marked independently. Also, the two examiners will not discuss a candidate's performance. Therefore, the candidate needs to be assured that poor performance in the first task is unlikely to influence the marks awarded in the second task.

Marking

The marking of all the stations is structured and thereby objective. This implies that irrespective of which examiner the candidates encounter, they are likely to obtain a similar score. Through the format of the MRCOG Part 3 examination, the RCOG ensures that each candidate is exposed to the same standard of the examination and all the candidates are evaluated against a similar standard.

Quality Assurance

The RCOG tries to ensure in every way that all parts of the membership examination are developed and delivered in a fair manner in accordance with the latest evidence-based research. In the part 3 examination, particular attention is given towards maintenance of consistency and secrecy between various examination circuits held for the MRCOG Part 3 examination. This is particularly important to ensure that the examination questions asked during a particular circuit do not leak out, thereby giving the candidates who are attempting the examination in the next circuit an unfair advantage. There may be numerous examination circuits for MRCOG examination, running simultaneously in the various centres (London, Singapore, Hong Kong, and Delhi) on each day of the examination.

Consistency is also important between the series of the examination held in May and November each year to ensure that both examination series approach similar level of difficulty. Prior to the examination, there is a careful checking process to ensure that all examination material is accurate, up-to-date, and evidence-based. Prior to the examination, the examiners undergo a training session to ensure that their marking is consistent and standardised for all the candidates. There is also a transparent appeals process for candidates who feel that they were unfairly marked for their performance during the examination.

CORE CLINICAL SKILLS DOMAINS

The five main core clinical skills domains which are tested in the MRCOG Part 3 examination include the following and are discussed briefly next.
1. Patient Safety (for detailed discussion, kindly refer to Chapter 4)
2. Communication with Patients (for detailed discussion, kindly refer to Chapter 5)
3. Communication with Colleagues (for detailed discussion, kindly refer to Chapter 6)
4. Information Gathering (for detailed discussion, kindly refer to Chapter 7)
5. Application of Knowledge (for detailed discussion, kindly refer to Chapter 8).

The candidate must keep in mind all these domains for every OSCE station, which they attempt. Each task is likely to assess a minimum of three core clinical skills domains. For each domain which is assessed, the examiner would be required to evaluate a candidate's performance as pass, borderline or fail. The examiner's judgement is converted into numerical scores, which is then used for calculating the candidate's mark. The candidate needs to understand that no single domain is more important than any other and the MRCOG Part 3 examination lays equal emphasis on the all the five domains.

The syllabus for the MRCOG defines the knowledge level expected for each part of the curriculum. However, some parts of the syllabus, which are commonly encountered in clinical practice, require significantly more in-depth knowledge in comparison to the others.[3] The standard expected for each question or task will be set on the basis of its difficulty level as well as how common it is in clinical practice. For example, the standard for a task relating to the management of common antenatal problem is likely to be higher than that for a task relating to precocious puberty.

CURRICULUM FOR MRCOG PART 3 EXAMINATION

The part 3 examination consists of 14 tasks, linked to one or more of the 14 knowledge-based modules (Table 2.1), which are part of the MRCOG Part 3 curriculum.[3] The candidates will be expected to demonstrate the application of their clinical knowledge of obstetrics and gynaecology through the following abilities:
- The candidates should be able to demonstrate a sound and comprehensive evidence-based understanding of the part 2 MRCOG curriculum in relation to the clinical tasks asked during the Part 3 examination.
- The candidates must be able to justify the investigations and interventions, which they think should be ordered for a particular patient.
- They should be able to critically interpret clinical findings and results of investigations and discuss the management plan.
- To be able to present a balanced view of the risks and benefits of various interventions.

In the part 3 examination, all 14 modules will be represented in every examination. According to changes in MRCOG examination pattern since September 2016, MRCOG Part 3 is an independent stand-alone examination, which tests the candidate's clinical knowledge and their application. In the previous examination pattern (prior to September 2016), the part 2 examination comprised of a written and oral examinations which shared a common outline. However, now as per the latest examination pattern, the part 3 is a stand-alone examination, which is set and marked completely independently. As a result, the candidates on each day of the examination are likely to have no prior knowledge regarding how each module may be tested. Each of the 14 modules will be tested with a separate task, so it is important for the candidates to revise all the required subject areas.

GOOD PRACTICE GUIDELINES

Patients should be able to trust doctors with their lives and health. According to the General Medical Council's (GMC) Good Practice Guidelines (2013), candidates must show respect for human life and make sure their practice meets the standards expected of them in following four domains so that their patients are able to trust them.[4]

TABLE 2.1: Knowledge-based modules in the UK obstetrics and gynaecology curriculum, which are tested in the MRCOG Part 3 examination.[3]

No. of module	Name of the module	Core skills tested
1	Teaching	*Communication with patients and families*: • Ability to demonstrate honesty where there is clinical uncertainty regarding surgical or management options • Using non-directional counselling when advising patients about various management options (including no treatment) *Communication with the colleagues*: • Ability to communicate with the colleague about the patient's clinical and operation notes legibly and with an ordered approach (date, time, patient identification details, etc.). • Demonstration of the ability to teach appropriate skills to other colleagues • Ability to prioritise which cases are urgent and which can be dealt with later or electively *Information gathering*: • Ability to take a concise and relevant antenatal history • Signposting and guiding the antenatal consultation • Ensuring that the patients understand the information provided to them • Ability to describe a clear action plan and the rationale for follow-up based on the discussion in case of an antenatal patient *Patient safety*: • Demonstration of the ability to triage patient to different patterns of antenatal care based on the risk factors • Demonstrating the awareness of safety of investigations and therapeutics during pregnancy (including safe prescribing) • Awareness regarding the issues of drug and alcohol abuse, domestic violence, and safeguarding the woman's rights • Understanding of clinical governance and risk management for women who refuse usual antenatal care *Application of clinical knowledge*: • Knowledge regarding antenatal care including pregnancy-induced hypertension (PIH), intrauterine growth restriction (IUGR), multiple gestation, preterm birth, prolonged pregnancy, vaginal birth after caesarean (VBAC), etc. • Ability to understand the findings and the results of clinical examination in the context of the clinical scenario • Awareness regarding the risks and benefits of various different management options, thereby balancing between the requirements of mother and foetus
2	Core surgical skills	*Communication with patients and families*: • Ability to demonstrate honesty where there is clinical uncertainty regarding surgical or management options • Using non-directional counselling when advising patients about various management options (including no treatment)

Contd...

Contd...

No. of module	Name of the module	Core skills tested
		Communication with colleagues: • Ability to communicate with the colleague about the patient's clinical and operation notes legibly and with an ordered approach (date, time, patient identification details, etc.) • Demonstration of the ability to teach appropriate skills to other colleagues • Ability to prioritise which cases are urgent and which can be dealt with later or electively *Information gathering*: • Demonstration of the understanding of essential preoperative investigations and significant clinical assessment • Ability to interpret clinical findings and investigations while making decision about surgical technique and approach • Ability to describe a clear action plan including ongoing management plan after a surgical procedure *Patient safety*: • Demonstrates understanding regarding principles of safe surgery including WHO safe surgery checklist • Demonstrates understanding of consent including consent of a child • Ability to assess an individual's mental capacity in relation to consent • Demonstrates the understanding of decision making and consent for patients lacking capacity • Demonstrates an understanding of moving and positioning the unconscious and recovering patient • Recognises limits of their clinical abilities • Demonstrates an understanding of when to call for help and involve senior colleagues and other disciplines *Application of clinical knowledge*: • Knowledge in relation to obstetric and gynaecological surgery including techniques and the risks and benefits of various procedures • Ability to critically appraise medical media in relation to surgical procedures • Is able to weigh up the pros and cons of surgical versus medical management of various clinical conditions • Understanding of the appropriate use of blood products
3	Post-operative care	*Communication with patients and families*: • Ability to provide psychological support to the patients and their family • Ability to discuss rehabilitation, discharge planning, recovery after discharge from hospital, return to work and follow-up • Ability to describe a clear and logical action plan and justification for follow-up after surgery *Communication with colleagues*: • Ability to diagnose post-operative complications • Formulating an appropriate post-operative management plan

Contd...

Contd...

No. of module	Name of the module	Core skills tested
		Information gathering: • Ability to request appropriate investigations and interpret those results • Summarises discussions concisely and checks at appropriate intervals that the patient is able to understand *Patient safety*: • Demonstrates an understanding of risk management and clinical governance processes in relation to post-operative complications • Recognises limits of their clinical abilities • Demonstration of an understanding regarding when to call for help and involve senior colleagues and other disciplines • Demonstrates an understanding of safe prescribing in post-operative care including recognition of drug interaction, allergies, and special circumstances, e.g. renal impairment *Application of clinical knowledge*: • Knowledge of management of the post-operative patient including fluid balance, analgesia, catheter management, and wound healing • Demonstrates understanding of the enhanced recovery programme and issues of post-operative rehabilitation • Demonstrate understanding regarding the early and late complications of surgery and their amendment
4	Antenatal care	*Communication with patients and families*: • Ability to tackle difficult or sensitive topics including domestic violence, drug, and alcohol abuse, child protection issues, female genital mutilation, etc. • Demonstration of honesty in cases of clinical uncertainty • Ability to discuss investigations, follow-up, and plan for antenatal care • Ability to concisely summarise discussions with antenatal patient *Communication with colleagues*: • Ability to discuss differential diagnosis or management plan for antenatal patients using a clear and logical approach with the colleagues • Discussing appropriate amount of details to ensure that the management plans are clear and easily understood by colleagues • Ability to communicate with colleagues in primary care GP (general practitioner), other specialties, e.g. obstetric anaesthetics and midwifery colleagues *Information gathering*: • Ability to take a concise and relevant antenatal history • Skills in signposting and guiding the antenatal consultation • Ensuring that the patient is able to understand what she is told and encouraging her to ask questions • Ability to describe to the antenatal patient a clear action plan and the rationale for follow-up based on the discussion

Contd...

Contd...

No. of module	Name of the module	Core skills tested
		Patient safety: • Triaging the patient to different patterns of antenatal care based on the risk factors • Demonstration of awareness regarding the safety of investigations and therapeutics during pregnancy including safe prescribing • Awareness of issues of drug and alcohol abuse, domestic violence, and safeguarding the patient's interests • Understanding of clinical governance and risk management for women who decline the usual antenatal care *Application of clinical knowledge*: • Knowledge of antenatal care including PIH, IUGR, multiple pregnancy, prolonged pregnancy, VBAC, preterm labour, etc. • Ability to interpret the findings and results of clinical examination and investigations in context of the clinical scenario • Developing awareness regarding the risks and benefits of various management options by balancing the requirements of mother and foetus
5	Maternal medicine	*Communication with patients and families*: • Ability to tackle sensitive topics including domestic violence and child protection issues • Demonstration of honesty in cases of clinical uncertainty • Providing information to the patient with coexisting medical disorders regarding both the impact of pregnancy on her pre-existing conditions as well as the impact of those conditions on the foetus *Communication with colleagues*: • Discussing differential diagnosis or management plan using a clear and logical approach for patients with both pre-existing medical disorders and those arising in pregnancy • Communication of adequate details to colleagues to ensure that the management plans are clear and easily understood by them • Communication with the colleagues in primary care (e.g. GP) and within the multidisciplinary team including nurse specialists, physicians, and psychiatrists *Information gathering*: • Ability to take a concise and relevant medical history • Skills in signposting and guiding the consultation • Ensuring that the patient is able to understand what is told to her and encouraging her to ask questions • Ability to describe a clear action plan and the rationale for follow-up based on the discussion to the patient with coexisting medical disorders *Patient safety*: • Demonstration of awareness regarding the safety of investigations and therapeutics during the pre-conception period, during pregnancy, and during the postnatal period including safe prescribing

Contd...

Contd...

No. of module	Name of the module	Core skills tested
		• Demonstrating an understanding regarding the impact of pregnancy on pre-existing conditions as well as the impact of those conditions on the foetus *Application of clinical knowledge*: • Demonstrating knowledge regarding the pre-conception, antenatal, and postnatal care including the risks of maternal morbidity and mortality related to the medical comorbidity
6	Management of labour	*Communication with patients and families*: • Ability to gain verbal or written consent for performing any intervention during labour or for operative delivery *Communication with colleagues*: • Ability to prioritise the cases requiring delivery based on the level of urgency • Demonstrating the understanding of various categories of caesarean deliveries • Ability of formulating an appropriate management plan for delivery • Demonstrates an understanding of the roles of the multidisciplinary team including liaison with laboratory colleagues in dealing with massive obstetric haemorrhage, liaison with neonatal team and other centres • Ability to communicate verbally with the multidisciplinary team including anaesthetists, theatre staff, and neonatologists in an efficient and timely manner • Demonstration of the ability to teach appropriate skills to other colleagues in a logical and coherent manner *Information gathering*: • Demonstration of ability to interpret notes on progress of labour, partogram, cardiotocography, and findings on vaginal examination in order to decide the appropriate management of delivery, both during the second and third stages • Ability to describe a clear action plan for management of delivery *Patient safety*: • Demonstrating the understanding regarding principles of safe surgery for operative delivery (including WHO safe surgery checklist) • Demonstrating appropriate prioritisation depending upon the urgency • Acknowledgment of medical error, omission or poor care. Apologizes, if appropriate • Demonstration of an understanding regarding the risk management and clinical governance processes in relation to management of delivery • Ability to critically appraise management of delivery in presence of complications *Application of clinical knowledge*: • Demonstration of knowledge regarding the management of delivery including pre-term delivery, management of malposition and malpresentation, and multiple pregnancy

Contd...

Contd...

No. of module	Name of the module	Core skills tested
		• Demonstration of clinical, technical, and operative skills • Demonstration of working knowledge regarding the roles and responsibilities of other members of the multidisciplinary team • Demonstration of understanding regarding neonatal networks and need to transfer to tertiary units
7	Management of delivery	*Communication with patients and families:* • Ability to gain verbal or written consent for intervention or operative delivery *Communication with colleagues:* • Ability to prioritise cases requiring urgent delivery • Understanding of the categories of caesarean delivery • Ability to formulate an appropriate management plan for delivery • Demonstrates an understanding regarding the roles of various members in the multidisciplinary team (e.g. coordination with laboratory colleagues in dealing with massive obstetric haemorrhage, coordination with neonatal team, etc.) • Ability to communicate verbally with the multidisciplinary team including anaesthetists, theatre staff, nursing staff, and neonatologists in an efficient and timely manner • Demonstrates ability to teach appropriate skills to other colleagues in a logical and coherent manner *Information gathering:* • Ability to interpret notes regarding progress of labour, partogram, cardiotocography, and findings on vaginal examination in order to decide the mode of delivery • Ability to clearly describe an action plan for management of delivery *Patient safety:* • Demonstrates understanding of principles of safe surgery for operative delivery (including WHO safe surgery checklist) • Demonstrates the ability to appropriately prioritise patients requiring delivery depending on the urgency • Acknowledgment of medical errors, omission or poor care • Demonstrates an understanding of risk management and clinical governance processes in relation to management of delivery • Ability to critically appraise management of delivery in presence of complications *Application of clinical knowledge:* • Adequate knowledge regarding management of delivery including pre-term delivery, management of malposition and malpresentation, and multiple pregnancy • Demonstration of appropriate clinical, technical, and operative skills • Demonstrates a working knowledge regarding the roles and responsibilities of other members in the multidisciplinary team • Understanding of neonatal networks and requirement for transfer to the tertiary units

Contd...

Contd...

No. of module	Name of the module	Core skills tested
8	Postpartum problems (the puerperium)	*Communication with patients and families:* • Ability to tackle difficult or sensitive topics including domestic violence, child protection issues, etc. • Demonstration of honesty in situations of clinical uncertainty • Ability to describe a clear action plan to the postpartum woman and the rationale for follow-up based on the discussion with her and her partner *Communication with colleagues:* • Devising a clear and logical approach to reach a differential diagnosis or management plan for postnatal patients • Communicating with colleagues an appropriate amount of detail to ensure management plans are clear and easily understood by colleagues • Ability to communicate with colleagues in primary care (e.g. GP), and other specialties, e.g. obstetric anaesthetics, neonatologists, physicians, microbiologists, midwifery colleagues, etc. *Information gathering:* • Ability to take a concise and relevant postnatal history • Skills in signposting and guiding the postnatal consultation • Ensuring the patient is able to understand what the doctor asks and encouraging her to ask questions • Ability to concisely summarise discussions with postnatal patient *Patient safety:* • Demonstration of awareness regarding the safety of various investigations and therapeutics during the postnatal period and lactation • Knowledge regarding safe prescribing • Understanding of safeguarding issues for neonates and vulnerable adults • Demonstrates understanding of psychological comorbidities, especially puerperal psychosis and risk of self-harm *Application of clinical knowledge:* • Demonstration of knowledge regarding postnatal care including the risks of maternal morbidity, mortality, and psychiatric disorders related to the postnatal period • Ability to recognise the critically ill or deteriorating postnatal patient and application of evidence-based approach for the management of postpartum complications
9	Gynaecological problems	*Communication with patients and families:* • Provides information to the patient regarding gynaecological abnormalities, investigations, and diagnoses and management of gynaecological problems • Describing a clear and logical action plan to the patient and rationale for follow-up

Contd...

Contd...

No. of module	Name of the module	Core skills tested
		Communication with colleagues: • Ability to prioritise cases appropriately depending on the level of urgency • Ability to describe the differential diagnosis and formulating an appropriate management plan *Information gathering:* • Demonstration of the ability to take a comprehensive history from patients and their families • Demonstrating a logical and clearly reasoned style of questioning • Ability to request appropriate investigations • Ability to interpret the results of various and operative findings in order to develop a clear management plan and rationale for follow-up • Summarises discussions concisely • Checks with the patient at appropriate intervals if she has understood what the doctor has told her *Patient safety:* • Demonstrating an understanding of risk management and clinical governance processes in relation to gynaecological disorders • Recognition of limits of their clinical abilities and demonstration of an understanding regarding when to call for help and involve senior colleagues • Demonstration of an understanding of safe prescribing in gynaecological disorders including recognition of drug interaction, allergies, and special circumstances, e.g. renal impairment • Demonstration of the understanding regarding the principles of safe surgery (including WHO safe surgery checklist) *Application of clinical knowledge:* • Demonstration of knowledge regarding the treatment of gynaecological disorders including menstrual disorders, endocrine disorders, disorders of puberty, congenital anomalies, menopause, and management of gynaecological emergencies • Demonstration of the ability to critically appraise medical media in relation to gynaecological treatment • Demonstrating the understanding regarding the role of imaging in gynaecological disorders • Understanding of referral pathways for gynaecological disorders • Demonstrating the ability to take informed consent including assessment of mental capacity • Demonstrating the ability to present various management options, along with their risks and benefits using non-directional counselling
10	Subfertility	*Communication with patients and families:* • Provision of information regarding infertility, investigations, and treatments in manageable amounts using patient friendly language, avoiding jargon

Contd...

Contd...

No. of module	Name of the module	Core skills tested
		• Demonstrates honesty around benefits, side effects, complications, and outcomes of fertility treatments • Demonstrates an understanding of the psychological needs of the partner as well as the infertile woman • Understanding of the psychological issues and sensitivities surrounding infertility *Communication with colleagues*: • Ability to describe the differential diagnosis • Formulation of an appropriate management plan *Information gathering*: • Ability to take a comprehensive history from both partners of an infertile couple • Ability to request suitable investigations • Ability to correctly interpret the results of investigations and operative findings from both female and male partners • Developing a clear management plan and rationale for follow-up • Ability to concisely summarise the discussions • Checking that the patient understands the information provided to her at appropriate intervals of time *Patient safety*: • Demonstrating an understanding regarding the risk management and clinical governance, and regulatory processes in relation to infertility (including the issues of confidentiality) • Understanding of the requirement to consider the welfare of the child while providing fertility treatments • Understanding of the risks of multiple pregnancy in association with fertility treatments *Application of clinical knowledge*: • Demonstration of knowledge regarding the treatment of infertility including surgical management of tubal disease, endometriosis, and male infertility • Demonstrating adequate evidence-based clinical knowledge regarding various assisted reproductive techniques such as ovulation induction, assisted conception, and gamete donation including the risks and limitations of these treatments • Demonstrating an ability to critically appraise medical media in relation to infertility treatments • Demonstrating an understanding regarding the role of the human fertilization and embryology association (HFEA) and the National Health Service funding restrictions and rationing of assisted conception • Understanding of the role of counselling for the infertile couple • Demonstrating the understanding of cultural issues as well as the issues relating to same sex partners and single parents

Contd...

Contd...

No. of module	Name of the module	Core skills tested
11	Sexual and reproductive health	*Communication with patients and families*: • Demonstration of tact, empathy, concern and respect for patients and maintenance of patient dignity at all times • Demonstration of a non-judgemental attitude while caring for patients • Demonstrating the ability to communicate with teenagers and encouraging them to involve their parents or guardians • Demonstrating respect for the patients' beliefs, values, and sexual diversity • Ability to describe an action plan in a clear and logical manner and rationale for follow-up *Communication with colleagues*: • Ability to appropriately prioritize the cases • Ability to describe the differential diagnosis and formulation of an appropriate management plan *Information gathering*: • Demonstration of the ability to take a comprehensive sexual health history • Ability to request appropriate investigations • Ability to interpret the results of the various investigations ordered and operative findings in order to develop a clear management plan and rationale for follow-up • Ability to concisely summarise discussions • Checking that the patient is able to understand what she is told at appropriate time intervals *Patient safety*: • Demonstration of an understanding regarding risk management and clinical governance processes in relation to sexual and reproductive health • Demonstrating an understanding of safe prescribing including recognition of drug interactions, allergies, and special circumstances, e.g. renal impairment *Application of clinical knowledge*: • Knowledge regarding sexual and reproductive health including contraception, UKMEC (UK Medical Eligibility Criteria) guidelines, unplanned pregnancy, and sexually transmitted infections (STIs) • Demonstration of understanding regarding the laws in relation to termination of pregnancy, STIs, consent, child protection, and the Sexual Offences Act 2003, etc. • Understanding regarding the roles and responsibilities of counsellors, police, primary care, social workers, genitourinary medicine (GUM) specialists, and the voluntary sector in the context of sexual and reproductive health
12	Early pregnancy care	*Communication with patients and families*: • Demonstration of empathic approach to the bereavement of early pregnancy loss • Ability to describe an action plan in a clear and logical manner and demonstrating a rationale for follow-up

Contd...

Contd...

No. of module	Name of the module	Core skills tested
		Communication with colleagues: • Demonstrates the ability to prioritise cases appropriately • Demonstrates the ability to describe the differential diagnosis and formulates an appropriate management plan *Information gathering*: • Demonstrates ability to take a comprehensive history from the patient • Demonstrates the ability to request appropriate investigations • Ability to interpret the results of those investigations and operative findings in order to develop a clear management plan and rationale for follow-up • Ability to concisely summarise discussions • Ability to check at appropriate intervals if the patient understands what has been told to her *Patient safety*: • Demonstration of an understanding regarding the risk management and clinical governance processes in relation to disorders of early pregnancy • Ability to recognise the limits of their clinical abilities • Demonstration of an understanding regarding when to call for help and involve senior colleagues • Demonstration of an understanding regarding safe prescribing in early pregnancy including recognition of drug interaction, allergies, and special circumstances, e.g. renal impairment • Demonstrates understanding of principles of safe surgery (including WHO safe surgery checklist) *Application of clinical knowledge*: • Demonstrates knowledge regarding early pregnancy complications including trophoblastic disease, ectopic pregnancy, and recurrent miscarriage • Demonstrates understanding regarding the surgical techniques for managing early pregnancy complications • Demonstration of an ability to critically appraise medical media in relation to early pregnancy disorders • Demonstration of the ability to present management options and their risks and benefits using non-directional counselling • Demonstration of an understanding regarding the impact of early pregnancy problems on future fertility and outcomes in future pregnancy
13	Gynaecological oncology	*Communication with patients and families*: • Provides information in manageable amounts to the patient and her family regarding investigations, diagnoses, and management of gynaecological malignancies • Demonstrates ability to deal sensitively with issues such as palliation and death • Ability to describe a clear and logical action plan • Understanding of the impact of gynaecological cancers and their treatment on future fertility and outcomes in future pregnancy

Contd...

Contd...

No. of module	Name of the module	Core skills tested
		Communication with colleagues: • Ability to prioritise the cases appropriately • Ability to describe the differential diagnosis and formulation of an appropriate management plan *Information gathering*: • Demonstrates ability to take comprehensive history from patients and their families • Ability to request appropriate investigations • Demonstrates the ability to interpret the results of those investigations and operative findings in order to develop a clear management plan and a rationale for follow-up • Demonstrates the ability to concisely summarise discussions • Ability to check with the patient at appropriate intervals if she is able to understand what has been told to her *Patient safety*: • Demonstrates an understanding regarding the referral pathways and targets for investigation and treatment of gynaecological cancers • Demonstrates an understanding of risk management and clinical governance processes in relation to gynaecological cancers • Ability to recognise limits of their clinical abilities • Demonstration of an understanding regarding when to call for help and involve senior colleagues • Demonstrates an understanding regarding safe prescribing in gynaecological cancers including recognition of drug interaction, allergies, and special circumstances, e.g. renal impairment • Demonstration of understanding regarding the principles of safe surgery (including WHO safe surgery checklist) *Application of clinical knowledge*: • Demonstration of knowledge regarding the epidemiology, presentation, investigation, treatment, and palliation of gynaecological malignancies • Demonstration of understanding regarding the roles and responsibilities of various members in the multidisciplinary team • Demonstration of an ability to critically appraise medical media in relation to gynaecological cancers • Demonstration of an understanding regarding the role of screening and imaging in gynaecological malignancies • Demonstrates understanding regarding the referral pathways for gynaecological cancers • Demonstrates ability to present various management options along with their risks and benefits using non-directional counselling
14	Urogynaecology and pelvic floor problems	*Communication with patients and families*: • Ability to provide information regarding urogynaecological examination, investigations, and treatment in manageable amounts using patient friendly language, avoiding jargon

Contd...

Contd...

No. of module	Name of the module	Core skills tested
		• Demonstration of honesty while explaining the benefits, side effects, complications, and clinical uncertainty related to the long-term outcomes of urogynaecological treatments
		• Demonstrates understanding of the psychological issues and sensitivities surrounding urogynaecological disorders and incontinence
		Communication with colleagues:
		• Demonstrates ability to describe the differential diagnosis and formulation of an appropriate management plan
		• Ability to clearly communicate the requirement and situation for the surgical management with the theatre staff, assistants, and the anaesthetists
		Information gathering:
		• Demonstration of the ability to take a comprehensive urogynaecological history
		• Demonstrates the ability to interpret urodynamic investigations, microbiological reports, cystometry, imaging, and fluid balance charts in order to reach a diagnosis and develop a management plan
		Patient safety:
		• Demonstrates an understanding regarding the principles of safe surgery (including WHO safe surgery checklist)
		• Demonstrates an understanding of safe prescribing in relation to urogynaecological therapeutics
		• Demonstrates an understanding regarding the contraindications and interactions of urogynaecological drugs and common medical treatments and their related comorbidities
		Application of clinical knowledge:
		• Demonstrates knowledge regarding the surgical, non-surgical, and medical management of urogynaecological disorders including pelvic organ prolapse, acute voiding disorders, overactive bladder, and stress urinary incontinence
		• Demonstration of an ability to critically appraise medical media in relation to urogynaecological treatments
		• Demonstration of an ability to weigh up pros and cons of surgical versus medical modalities for the management of urogynaecological disorders

Source: Royal College of Obstetricians and Gynaecologists. (2017). Part 3 MRCOG: syllabus. [online] Available from https://www.rcog.org.uk/en/careers-training/mrcog-exams/part-3-mrcog-exam/part-3-mrcog-syllabus/ [Accessed July 2017].

1. Knowledge, Skills, and Performance

The candidates must ensure that the care of the patients remains their first concern. They must demonstrate good standard of practice and care by keeping their professional knowledge and skills up to date. They must work within the limits of their competence.

2. Safety and Quality

The candidate (doctor) must take prompt action if they think that the patient's safety, dignity or comfort is being compromised. They must take steps to protect and promote the health of their patients.

3. Communication, Partnership, and Teamwork

The candidate must demonstrate good communication skills by treating the patients as individuals and respecting their dignity. They must treat patients politely and considerately and respect their right to confidentiality. The doctors must work in partnership with patients by listening and respond to their concerns and preferences. They must remain professional and in control of the consultation.

As the candidates enter the examination booth, they must introduce themselves to the actor and address her or him by name. In case both a role-player and an examiner are present at a station, the candidate must only interact with the role-player, but not with the examiner. Towards the end, the candidates can ask the examiners if they have any questions for them.

The candidate must provide information to the role-player in a manner they would be able to understand. As far as possible all medical jargon must be avoided. It is a good idea to summarise the information back to the role-player to ensure that the candidate has fully understood the information imparted by the role-player. No matter what decision the patient takes regarding their management, the doctor must respect the patient's right to reach decisions regarding their care and treatment. They must ask the patient or role-player if they have understood their questions to ensure that the patient has been able to completely comprehend them. Communication with the patients has been discussed in details in Chapter 5.

On some OSCE stations, the candidates may be required to demonstrate their communication skills while interacting with their colleagues. They must show that they are capable of working in partnership with their colleagues in a way that best serves their patients' interests. Communication with the colleagues has been best discussed in Chapter 6.

4. Maintaining Trust

Candidate must be able to demonstrate honesty and act with integrity in order to build the trust of their patients. The doctors are personally accountable for their professional practice and must always be prepared to justify their decisions and actions.

PREPARATION FOR AN OSCE EXAMINATION

Preparing for an OSCE examination varies from that preparing for a theory examination. The OSCE examination tests clinical and communication skills rather than pure theoretical knowledge. Marks are awarded for each task. Hence, it is essential for the candidate to divide their time so as they are able to perform all the tasks.

These skills tested during the MRCOG Part 3 examination are fundamental to high quality patient care, and have been proposed by the GMC's Good Practice Guidelines (2013). These four duties expected of any doctor registered with the GMC include 'Knowledge, skills, and performance'; 'Safety and quality'; 'Communication, partnership, and teamwork'; and 'Maintaining trust'. These have been discussed in details previously in the text.

The candidate's theoretical knowledge has already been tested in MRCOG Part 2 examination. Therefore it is a good idea to immediately attempt the Part 3 MRCOG examination after clearing the part 2 examination, while the candidate is still fresh with the theoretical knowledge. Depending upon their personal situation and the time they can devote for examination preparation, candidate may require anywhere between 1 month to 6 months to prepare for MRCOG Part 3 examination.

Part 3 MRCOG examination is not about knowledge; rather it is about communication skills. Since the candidates who are attempting the part 3 examination have already passed the Part 2 MRCOG, they already have the best of knowledge. They just need to apply their clinical knowledge in the part 3 examination.

OSCE stations can be practiced with a small group of colleagues, where one person can act as the candidate, second one as the role-player, third one as an examiner who is observing and marking the candidate. Another person can time the entire scenario to ensure that the candidate completes the entire scenario within 10 minutes. Through this set-up, the candidate would be able to get a feel of working under pressure, where he/she has to complete the entire scenario within 10 minutes like in a real examination.

If it is not possible to practice in a group, the candidate needs to at least practice with an examination buddy who can act as a role-player. The candidate can practice with a layman (candidate's sibling or good friend), who does not have a medical background. Role-players scripts are given in this book as well as in other books on OSCE stations. The exam buddy should be advised to give an honest feedback to the candidate. If a non-medico likes the candidate's communication style, the candidate can be self-assured that they are going on the right track. They must carefully listen to the layman's feedback while practicing. The candidate can record the entire scenario in a video and later watch the video to carefully note their own expressions and actions.

REFERENCES

1. Royal College of Obstetricians and Gynaecologists. (2017). Part 3 MRCOG exam. [online] Available from https://www.rcog.org.uk/en/careers-training/mrcog-exams/part-3-mrcog-exam/ [Accessed July 2017].
2. Harden RM, Stevenson M, Downie WW, et al. Assessment of clinical competence using objective structured examination. Br Med J. 1975;1(5955):447-51.
3. Royal College of Obstetricians and Gynaecologists. (2017). Part 3 MRCOG: syllabus. [online] Available from https://www.rcog.org.uk/en/careers-training/mrcog-exams/part-3-mrcog-exam/part-3-mrcog-syllabus/ [Accessed July 2017].
4. General Medical Council. (2013). Good medical practice (2013). [online] Available from http://www.gmc-uk.org/guidance/good_medical_practice.asp [Accessed July 2017].

3

Tips for the Examination

INTRODUCTION

The MRCOG Part 3 examination is more than just the test of the candidate's clinical knowledge. This examination is also the test of candidate's ability to work under stress, candidate's communication skills, and ability to counsel and satisfy the patient. Since this is a difficult and an important examination, the candidates need to develop some strategies to help them with the examination. This chapter would be describing some tips which the candidates must master in order to sail through the examination.

GENERAL INFORMATION

As described previously in Chapter 2, there are 14 tasks in a circuit, where each task is based on one of the 14 modules detailed in the syllabus. Each task is for 12 minutes in length, inclusive of 2 minutes of the initial reading time. There are two types of tasks in the part 3 examination: simulated patient or colleague task (interaction with an actor who has been trained and instructed to carry out the role, she/he is to play) and structured discussion tasks (direct interaction with the clinical examiner). A trained clinical examiner would be present on all the 14 tasks, whereas a lay examiner along with a clinical examiner would be present on 4 out of the 14 tasks.

To allow for more in-depth assessment of the candidate's applied clinical knowledge, sometimes 'linked or preparatory tasks', may be present in a circuit. There may also be stations where candidates are required to undertake some writing task.

As previously explained, linked task is one where the second task is connected to the first. For example, the candidate may be given some time to prepare some task and then discuss this with a role-player or an examiner at the next station. The task involved could include writing a protocol, preparing an audit, criticizing an information leaflet, etc. and explaining them to the clinical examiner on the next station. The candidate may also be required to counsel the role player regarding some information which she downloaded from the internet.

Time Required For Preparation

Obviously the candidates attempting the part 3 examination have already cleared their part 2 examination. Therefore, these candidates have already demonstrated the core clinical knowledge about the subject, which is tested by the part 2 examinations. They now need to demonstrate their core clinical skills by clearing the part 3 examination. The clinical knowledge, which the candidates had acquired while preparing for the part 2 examination, is still likely to be fresh in their minds. Therefore, it is important that they try to attempt the part 3 examination as soon as possible. However, during this time they are likely to have their family and work commitments. Most of the candidates are likely to be practicing in the hospital at this time. Also, most of the candidates would also have commitments related to the families and kids. Therefore, the candidates need to plan according. Approximately 6 months of preparation time should be sufficient for most of the candidates. During the initial months of preparation, it would be sufficient to devote about 4–6 hours every day for the examination. However, in last 1–2 months before the examination, it is advisable to take leave from work and devote time exclusively towards the preparation for part 3.

ADVICE FOR THE EXAMINATION

Being Natural and not Taking Stress

The candidates must not panic rather they must treat the part 3 examination as a routine day in the antenatal clinic, gynaecology clinic, labour ward or being on call for emergencies, where they are applying their clinical knowledge and thinking about patient safety in every decision they make. The candidates must try to remain as natural as possible. While treating the patients in the clinics, the doctors are often talking to patients and colleagues, taking their history and gathering relevant information. These are the very skills, which would be assessed in the part 3 examination, so if the candidates mentally practice these skills on a daily basis in the clinics, they are likely to have little problem in passing this examination.

Also, the MRCOG Part 3 examination is aimed at the level of an ST5 (specialist trainee) trainee. ST5 level means a UK trainee who has completed 5 years of structured training, is able to manage the majority of problems encountered on the delivery suite, is able to tackle most common gynaecological emergencies, and is able to run general gynaecological and antenatal clinics with minimal or indirect supervision. At this level, the candidate is not expected to be an expert yet. Therefore, during the MRCOG Part 3 examination, the candidate must remember to inform the consultant, keeping in mind the aspect of patient safety, as they would have normally done in their clinical practice.

Though there is nothing wrong in calling for senior support, the candidate must remember 'not to call the consultant for everything' because that is likely to demonstrate under confidence on part of the candidate. Many candidates are not aware about the structure of National Healthcare Services in the UK. This is especially important for the overseas candidates who have never practiced in the UK. It is, therefore, important for a candidate to have practiced in the UK healthcare system before attempting the part 3 examination. Even if they have never worked in the UK, it is essential that the candidates understand the structure of healthcare system, the concept of clinical governance and its application in the clinical practice in terms of evidence-based practice, green top guidelines, incident reporting, audit, concept of risk management, etc. It is also important for the candidates to understand the role of midwives, specialist nurses, multidisciplinary team, and allied health professionals in the UK healthcare practice.

Reading the Question Carefully

To spend time in carefully reading the question may appear to be a basic advice but this is really very important. If the task requires a candidate to take history as well as counselling the patient, the candidates must distribute their time equally between taking history and counselling her. On the other hand, if the station requires the candidates to only counsel the patient, they must not waste their time in taking an elaborate history. Usually, there is more than one task which the candidate is expected to perform. The candidate must remember to cover all the tasks within the stipulated time.

The candidate tasks may provide the candidates with a clue regarding what they are expected to do. Words like 'explain' or 'justify' help in indicating the skills, which the candidate is expected to demonstrate. Therefore it is extremely important for the candidates to carefully read the tasks which they are expected to perform.

The candidates are given 2 minutes to read the scenario before each task starts. The first time the candidate reads through the information posted on the outside of the booth, they should focus on the clinical scenario. Mentally they should recollect the clinical knowledge related to that clinical scenario. They should read the candidate instructions again, this time focusing on the tasks they would be required to perform. Now the candidates must decide their strategic approach for dealing with the station and think about the domains which the station would be covering.

Facing the Examiner and the Role-Player

In the stations with structured viva, there would only be an examiner whose questions the candidate is expected to answer. In a structured viva, the candidates are not expected to introduce themselves. They can just smile, greet the examiner, and sit down. The examiner will direct the candidate in the beginning of the task asking them relevant questions on the way.

In case of a task with a simulated patient, both the examiner and the role-player or actor would be present at the booth. The candidate needs to adopt a friendly approach in such kinds of stations. They would need to introduce themselves by name and check up with the patient how they would like to be addressed, i.e. whether it would be alright to address her by her first name? The candidate must also focus on the nonverbal aspects of their communication. In most situations a friendly smile is likely to be appropriate. However, if the candidate is going to be breaking bad news, they must demonstrate sensitivity right from the very beginning of the scenario.

Approaching the Role-Player

Some general skills which the candidate must follow while approaching the role-player are described in Box 3.1.[1]

Carefully Observing and Listening to the Role-Player

In the stations with a simulated patient or a simulated clinical colleague, the actor involved would have been carefully instructed about the scenario and would be provided with some structured questions to ask the candidate. These questions are designed to guide the candidate in such a way that they are able to address all the domains which they need to pass the various tasks which they perform. Therefore, the candidate must not only carefully listen to the role-player's questions, but also carefully observe their body language and expressions. In case the candidate is going off the track, role-player would be giving indirect clues to help the candidate. For example, if a role player continuously keeps crying while the candidate is taking her history, it may be a warning sign that the candidate has missed some important aspect of the history. Therefore, the candidates must carefully listen to the role-player and if the role-player asks a question, particularly if they repeat the question, then the candidate must take the clue that role-player is directing them in a particular direction. The role players usually try to help the candidates and prevent the discussion moving into an irrelevant area.

Practice with an Exam Buddy and a Stop Clock

While preparing for the part 3 examination, the candidates must preferably practice with the help of their exam buddy. The examination buddy could be

---

BOX 3.1: Skills to be followed while approaching the role-player.[1]

- The candidates must greet the role-player and then introduce themselves
- They must avoid the use of medical jargon
- They must establish eye contact with the role-player
- They must keep a pleasant and warm expression on their face
- They must listen carefully to the role-player without any interruption
- They must invite questions from the role-player
- At the end of conversation, the candidate must summarise what the role-player has told them
- Candidate must maintain an appropriate demeanour while conveying empathy, concern, and attention at the time the role players are telling their problems or concerns
- Candidate must avoid any visible display of the signs of nervousness (e.g. repeatedly glancing at one's watch)

their friend, spouse, sibling or colleague, who would play the role of the patient. While practicing with their examination buddy, the candidates must preferably time their practice sessions so that they get well acquainted in answering the questions within the stipulated time.

Use of Props

If there is presence of some props on the OSCE station, the candidates must make use of them. The equipment may be particularly present on the teaching stations; for example, the candidate may find a doll and model of a pelvis for teaching breech delivery, or a pair of forceps or vacuum equipment (e.g. Kiwi® cups) for teaching instrumental vaginal delivery. If the equipment is present on the station, the examiner would be expecting the candidate to use the equipment for demonstrating their ideas. This is especially the case when there is a teaching task with a simulated junior colleague. In such cases the candidate must also give a chance to the simulated junior colleague to hold and use the given props. Only this way the simulated candidate would be able to demonstrate whether they have correctly understood what they had been taught. This step is essential for the candidate to pass the station. It is also important that the candidate shows the correct use of the props to the simulated junior colleague. If they themselves use the props incorrectly, they are unlikely to pass the station.

Drawings

At the start of the examination, the candidates are usually provided with a notepad and pencil to take with them while they are moving across several stations. They can use this notepad for taking brief notes if required or they can use it for making small diagrams through which they can explain the anatomical details and various pathologies to the role-player.

Avoiding the Use of Medical Jargon

The candidates must take care to avoid using medical terminology while talking to the role-player who is simulating a patient.[2] It is important for the candidate to ensure that the role-player understands everything they are explaining to them, especially while counselling, breaking bad news or explaining the diagnosis or the management plan. For example, it is reasonable to use the word 'womb' instead of uterus or down below instead of vulva when speaking to patients. It does not really matter what kind of terminology the candidate uses, the main concern is that the role-player or the patient should clearly understand what they are being explained.

On the other hand, while talking to the role-player who is playing the role of a simulated colleague, the candidate can usually use medical terminology similar to what they would in a real life scenario. However, still the candidate needs to ensure that the role-player understands what has been told to them.

Strength

Personal strength, mental more than physical, is important in order to sustain through this difficult examination. Giving this 3-hours long examination (without any gaps or breaks) in itself is hard work. Though it may sound strange the candidates must be well prepared to deal with the adverse situations, which may seriously affect their performance on the day of the examination. They must also take care of trivial details such as having a good sleep on the night before the examination, trying to remain as stress free and relaxed as possible prior to the examination, ensuring that they reach the examination centre on time, etc. It is especially important for the overseas candidates to consider staying overnight at a place close to the examination centre rather than rushing in for a long-distance travel, early on the morning of the examination. The candidate should remain calm and stress free on the morning of the examination. They should preferably avoid any last-minute revision on the morning of examination. The part 3 examination is the test of candidate's core clinical skills. Therefore, cramming just prior to the examination is unlikely to help. Another practical advice which the candidates must take into consideration prior to the examination is to ensure that they are not overly tired on the day of the examination. It is best to take a few weeks off prior to the examination. In case this is not possible, the candidates must at least ensure that they are not on-call duty on the day before the examination. They should also not stay up late on the night before the examination. Other practical aspects which the candidate must take care of include having a light but nutritious breakfast or lunch prior to the examination and wearing comfortable, but formal or professional clothes for the examination. The candidates do not need to bring the white doctors coat for the examination.

Since the MRCOG Part 3 examination is a postgraduate level examination, it requires at least 6 months for preparation. This would be a hard work because simultaneously most of the candidates would be involved in clinical work in the hospital and the clinics. During this time, it is important that the candidates take good care of themselves. They must have a healthy diet and get involved in some exercise activity on a regular basis. The best form of exercise could be walking on a regular basis, cycling or swimming. Getting involved in some sports activity of one's choice (e.g. 1 hour of tennis every day) may also help. As far as possible, the candidates must avoid the use of stimulants such as nicotine, caffeine, alcohol, etc. to help them improve their performance.

Despite the fact that one needs to concentrate solely on academics while preparing for this examination, friends and family must not be completely ignored. Maintenance of work–life balance is of utmost importance.

It is also essential to get a sufficient amount of sleep every day. Adequate amount of sleep is essential for good retention of facts and memory. Avoid cramming for the examination by using stimulants like caffeine to keep you awake and revising into the early hours of the morning.

Adequate sleep forms an important aspect of one's learning and memory. Animal and human research studies have indicated that sleep helps in promoting learning and memory in two distinctive ways:

1. A sleep-deprived person is incapable of concentrating in the best possible way and therefore is not able to learn efficiently.
2. Sleep, especially the rapid eye movement (REM) sleep, itself has a role in the consolidation of memory, which is important for registering new information.[3]

Studying continuously at a stretch is usually not recommended. It is a good idea to take small breaks in between every hour of studies. However, the candidate must ensure that break does not become very long otherwise it may become difficult to re-establish the study pace. This short break can be utilized for eating or drinking something or making a short phone call or spending time with your pet.

Resources for Studying

With new advancements in the speciality of obstetrics and gynaecology, the clinicians need to keep themselves abreast with the changes especially those occurring in the arena of evidence-based medicine. New guidelines and developments keep getting published and the clinicians attempting the part 3 examination need to be up-to-date with these developments. Therefore, they need to resort to those resources which would keep them well informed. Some of those resources are as follows:

- *RCOG Green-top Guidelines*: Present both the summary guidance and the evidence levels for each statement.[4]
- *NICE (National Institute for Health and Care Excellence) guidelines*: An excellent resource providing a very detailed discussion regarding the evidence that reinforces the guidance.[5]
- *RCOG's CPD (Continuing Professional Development) journal, TOG (The Obstetrician and Gynaecologist) articles*: Evidence-based reviews of practice, including ethical and clinical governance topics.[6]
- Scientific impact statements.
- Clinical governance advice, good practice documents, consent advice, and patient information leaflets.[7]
- The Lindsay Stewart Committee for audit and clinical informatics delivers audits and clinical improvement projects on behalf of the RCOG: this can be accessed from the website https://www.rcog.org.uk/en/about-us/governance/committees/lindsay-stewart-committee-for-audit-and-clinical-informatics/[8]
- Reviews, Clinical Governance, and Ethics Resources.
- *The Cochrane Library (www.cochranelibrary.com)*: An online resource containing systematic reviews and meta-analyses of research for numerous clinical conditions. The guidelines are powerfully evidence-based and provide detailed protocols regarding the practice of clinical medicine.
- *Recently published research papers published in the major peer-reviewed journals*: These include journals such as the British Journal of Obstetrics and Gynaecology, Lancet, and New England Journal of Medicine.
- *Textbooks*: Textbooks may be essential to brush up one's knowledge in clinical sciences, which are usually asked in the part 1 examination.

This is usually not required for part 2 or part 3 examination. However, if the candidates feel that they have a gap in knowledge and they need to refresh their knowledge, they must read the relevant textbooks.

- *Attending preparatory courses*: The candidates can attend the preparatory course for MRCOG Part 3 examination organized by the RCOG.

In-depth Knowledge about the Subject

Though the part 3 examination aims at testing the candidate's core clinical skills and is about communication abilities, to be able to correctly manage and treat them, the candidates need to have an in-depth knowledge about the subject. The candidates' one-point resource for revision is the core curriculum on the RCOG website. The candidates may find the e-learning resources in StratOG (https://stratog.rcog.org.uk) to be really useful. The candidates, especially the overseas candidates, must be aware about the working in the UK healthcare system. They must be particularly aware about the concept of clinical governance as well as the various UK laws like the Mental Capacity Act, the Abortion Act, Lord Fraser competency, illegal practice of female genital mutilation, etc.

REFERENCES

1. Sloan DA, Donnelly MB, Schwartz RW, et al. The Objective Structured Clinical Examination. The new gold standard for evaluating postgraduate clinical performance. Ann Surg. 1995;222(6):735-42.
2. Graham S, Brookey J. Do Patients Understand? Perm J. 2008 Summer;12(3): 67-9.
3. Eugene AR, Masiak J. The Neuroprotective Aspects of Sleep. Medtube Sci. 2015;3(1):35-40.
4. Royal College of Obstetricians and Gynaecologists. (2017). Guidelines. [online] Available from https://www.rcog.org.uk/guidelines [Accessed November 2017].
5. National Institute for Health and Care Excellence. NICE guidance. [online] Available from https://www.nice.org.uk/guidance [Accessed November 2017].
6. Royal College of Obstetricians and Gynaecologists. (2017). TOG. [online] Available from https://www.rcog.org.uk/en/guidelines-research-services/tog/ [Accessed November 2017].
7. Patient access. (2017). Making lives better. [online] Available from https://patient.info/in [Accessed November 2017].
8. Royal College of Obstetricians and Gynaecologists. (2017). Lindsay Stewart Committee for Audit and Clinical Informatics. [online] Available from https://www.rcog.org.uk/en/about-us/governance/committees/lindsay-stewart-committee-for-audit-and-clinical-informatics/ [Accessed November 2017].

4

Patient Safety

INTRODUCTION

Patient safety can be considered as a subject area, highlighting safety in healthcare practice through the prevention, reduction, recording, and evaluation of medical errors which may be responsible for producing adverse events. The Institute of Medicine (IOM) has defined patient safety as 'the prevention of harm to patients.'[1] According to the IOM, patient safety can be considered to be indistinguishable from the delivery of quality healthcare. Some practices which can be included in the category of patient safety practices include appropriate use of prophylaxis to prevent venous thromboembolism (VTE) in patients at risk, appropriate use of antibiotic prophylaxis in surgical patients to prevent post-operative infections, etc.[2] Measures for patient safety help in reducing the rate of infections, help in prevention of mistakes, and ensure strong lines of communication between the hospital, patients, and their families.

An important aspect of patient safety is dealing with the patient's complaints. Despite of clinicians' best efforts towards patients' safety, things may sometimes go wrong resulting in the patient's complaints. According to Patients Association (2013), a complaint can be defined as '*an expression of dissatisfaction made to an organisation, either written or spoken, and whether justified or not, requiring a response*'[3] Communication failure can be considered as the most common cause of the patient's complaints. In the department of obstetrics and gynaecology, complaints are most commonly encountered in the postnatal period. It is important for the doctors practicing in the NHS to effectively deal with the patients complaints as demonstrated in Flow chart 4.1.

PRIORITISATION

One method of ensuring patient safety is the ability to correctly prioritise the patients depending on their level of urgency. OSCE (Objective Structured

Flow chart 4.1: Algorithm for dealing with patient's complaints.

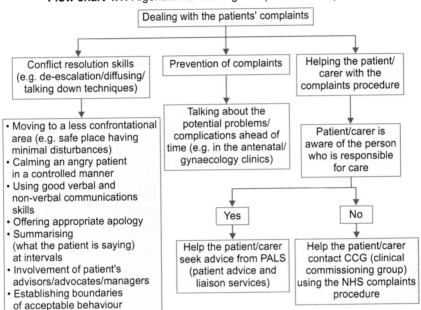

Clinical Examination) stations pertaining to prioritisation may check the doctor's ability to set priorities in their clinical work. The clinical scenarios may involve a candidate to prioritise between a busy labour ward, and the calls they may receive from the ward or the rest of the hospital. It may also involve setting up the priorities in the operating list. It is important to be familiar with waiting times, such as target referrals for suspected cancers. For example, once the diagnosis of cancer has been made, then there is a 31-day target to commence treatment.[4]

OSCE STATION 1: VAGINAL BIRTH AFTER CAESAREAN SECTION

Candidate's Instructions

A 34-year-old schoolteacher, in her third pregnancy, the previous two having been delivered by caesarean section, presents at 37 weeks' gestation requesting for a trial of vaginal delivery in the antenatal clinic. You are the registrar on duty, who would be assessing her. The task is for 12 minutes (inclusive of 2 minutes of reading time). You have 10 minutes to counsel her about the situation. You shall be awarded marks for the following tasks:

Candidate's tasks:

- Take the relevant history from the patient
- How will you counsel her about her request?
- What precautions will you take to ensure a safe vaginal delivery?

These tasks cover the domains as discussed next.

Core Clinical Skills Domains

Core clinical skills domains tested:
• Patient safety • Communication with patients • Information gathering • Application of knowledge.

Module Tested

The module tested in this station is Module 7 or 'The Management of Delivery'.

Role-player's Brief

You are Mary Grant, a 34-year-old married schoolteacher. This is your third pregnancy. Your previous two pregnancies were via caesarean delivery. Your first child is now a 7-year-old boy. He was delivered by caesarean delivery because there was no progress in labour. Your second pregnancy was also by caesarean section because the baby's heart rate started dipping. Your second child is now a 4-year-old girl, Ann. During both the caesarean deliveries, you had no complications at the time of surgery or during the post-operative period.

You have now reached 37 weeks of gestation. Your present pregnancy has largely been uneventful and you had been getting regular check-ups done. You have heard from your friends that vaginal birth gives a real feeling of motherhood. You are therefore adamant that you want a vaginal birth in this pregnancy.

Prompt Questions

- Is vaginal birth possible in my case?
- Do I necessarily require a caesarean section in this delivery?
- Is vaginal birth after two previous caesarean deliveries successful?
- Is vaginal birth after two previous caesarean deliveries associated with any complications?

EXAMINER'S INSTRUCTIONS AND STRUCTURED MARK SHEET

The examiner will mark the candidate on the basis of various tasks which are allotted to the candidate. Out of a total score of 20, the examiner can award a maximum of 18 marks, which are distributed between various candidate tasks as shown next. The role-player can award a maximum of 2 marks to the candidate. Each candidate task must be globally scored by the examiner.

Taking the Relevant History from the Patient

- What was the cause for the previous two caesarean deliveries?
- Was it a recurrent cause? [If the previous caesarean deliveries were performed due to a recurrent problem (e.g. contracted pelvis or a congenital malformation of the uterus), vaginal delivery would be unsafe for her].
- Are previous notes of caesarean section available with the patient?

- Type of previous caesarean section—if classical or inverted-T incisions (Figs. 4.1 and 4.2), unsafe for trial of vaginal delivery.
- Did she experience any complications (especially infection) during the post-operative period during each pregnancy? (Post-operative infection, especially during the second caesarean section is likely to result in scar weakness).
- Did she experience any complications in the present pregnancy (e.g. placenta praevia, transverse lie, etc.), which may require a compulsory caesarean delivery during this pregnancy.
- Why does she want a vaginal delivery in this pregnancy?

Marking Scheme

0	1	2	3	4	5	6
Fail		Borderline		Pass		

Counselling about her Request

- The patient should be counselled about the risk related to the trial of vaginal delivery.
- The patient must be warned about the potential risks of uterine rupture, requirement of an emergency caesarean section, and other complications associated with trial of vaginal birth.
- There may be a requirement of an emergency caesarean delivery. The complications of emergency caesarean section should be discussed, including requirement of a hysterectomy in case the uterus ruptures. Where there is a rupture, there is a possibility of foetal bradycardia or a drop in the baby's heart rate.
- Part of the counselling in such a patient should include the problems that could arise when the pregnancy goes post-term. Induction of labour with

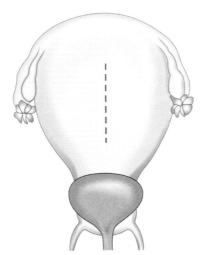

Fig. 4.1: Classical incision in the upper uterine segment.

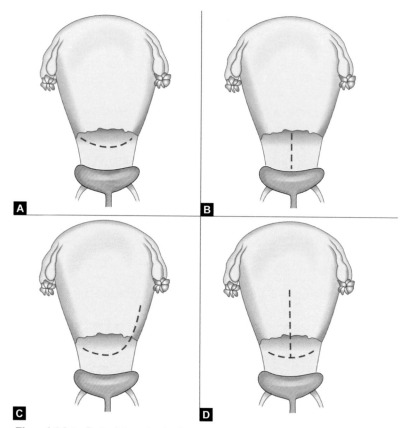

Figs. 4.2A to D: Incisions in the lower uterine segment: (A) Low transverse incision; (B) Low vertical incision; (C) J-shaped incision, and (D) T-shaped incision.

prostaglandins is relatively contraindicated in this patient due to the risk of scar rupture. Also, no oxytocics must be used during labour. If the patient goes post-term, an elective caesarean section is likely to be the preferred mode of delivery. In addition, if the patient went into labour and required augmentation, Syntocinon® would be relatively unsafe because of the risk of rupture. In this case, again, caesarean section is likely to be a safer option.

Marking Scheme

0	1	2	3	4	5	6
Fail		Borderline		Pass		

Ensuring the Safety of Vaginal Delivery

- Mandatory hospital confinement
- Blood should be sent for grouping and save or cross-matching. Complete blood count (including haemoglobin and haematocrit levels) be done.
- To ensure the safety of her baby, continuous foetal heart monitoring would be done during labour.

- There would be preparations for emergency caesarean delivery in case it is required.

Marking Scheme

0	1	2	3	4	5	6
Fail		Borderline		Pass		

Role-player's Score

The role-player can award a maximum of 2 marks to the candidate.

Marking Scheme

0	1	2
Role-player never wants to see candidate again	Role-player prepared to see candidate again	Role-player happy to see candidate again

Total score: /20

DISCUSSION

Issues

Traditional practice being followed at most centres indicates that a woman with previous two or more caesarean deliveries must be delivered by caesarean section in their next delivery due to an increased risk of uterine rupture during labour in these women. Progressively, this method has been interrogated because there are no randomised trials to rationalise the reason to follow this approach. In fact, the available research studies have shown that the risk of uterine rupture with vaginal delivery in case of a woman with two or more previous caesarean scars is similar to that in women with one previous caesarean section.[5-8] This delivery should, however, take place only in the hospital where there are facilities for emergency delivery in case of failure of vaginal birth and suitable expertise is available. Also each case needs to be individualised because some women (e.g. history of previous successful vaginal delivery, those women where the caesarean delivery was not performed due to a recurrent cause, absence of any indication for caesarean delivery in the present pregnancy, absence of post-operative scar infection during previous surgeries, etc.) are likely to be associated with an increased success rate in comparison to women with no such factor.[9] Therefore, before offering this choice to the patient, careful consideration must be given to her past obstetric history and the current pregnancy. It is only after appropriate counselling about the risks that this option should be allowed.

Pitfalls

The major mistake which a candidate can commit in such type of station is arguing about the complications of vaginal delivery with the patient and forcing her to adopt the option of caesarean section.

Variations

Various variations which could be present in this type of station include maternal request for caesarean delivery during her first pregnancy or request for caesarean delivery and not vaginal delivery following one previous caesarean delivery.

OSCE STATION 2: MANAGEMENT OF RECURRENT URINARY INCONTINENCE AFTER SUCCESSFUL SURGERY

Candidate's Instructions

You are the registrar on duty who has to attend Mrs Joan Dunn, a 65-year-old woman, who has returned to the urogynaecology clinic with the complaints of recurrent urinary incontinence 4 years after a successful colposuspension. There are no significant findings on general and pelvic examination.

The task is for 12 minutes (inclusive of 2 minutes of reading time). You have 10 minutes to talk to her about the situation. You shall be awarded marks for the following tasks:

Candidate's tasks:

- Take the relevant history from the patient
- What investigations would you carry out in such patient?
- Devise a subsequent management plan for her.

These tasks cover the domains as discussed next.

Core Clinical Skills Domains

Core clinical skills domains tested:

- Patient safety
- Communication with patients
- Information gathering
- Application of knowledge.

Module Tested

The module tested in this station is Module 14 or 'Urogynaecology and Pelvic Floor Problems.'

Role-player's Brief

You are Mrs Joan Dunn, a 65-year-old woman, a part-time learning support assistant. You have been experiencing leaking of urine since past month. The leaking does not occur all the time and typically occurs only when you are laughing, coughing, sneezing or running. There has also been an increased frequency of passing urine 8–10 times a day. There is history of nocturia, and you have to wake up about 2–3 times during the night to pass urine. However, there is no history of bedwetting. There is no history of urgency, you are able to hold your desire to pass urine until you reach the toilet. There have been no accidents related to passage of urine in the past because you were able to reach the toilet on time. There has been no history of burning sensation or pain while passing urine.

- You were perfectly normal 4 years back, following which had started first experiencing these symptoms. You underwent a surgery at that time because your symptoms were quite severe. You do not have the surgery notes with you, but you remember the doctor telling you that the surgery would help supporting the urethra to help keep it closed, while you cough and sneeze. Your symptoms greatly improved following surgery and you had been facing no problems since last 4 years, except last 1 month, when your symptoms have recurred again.
- You went through the menopause at age the age of 47 years and there have been no gynaecological problems since then.
- You have had two children, both normal deliveries and all weighing over 3 kg.
- You remain sexually active.
- There is no other significant history. You are non-alcoholic and non-smoker. You occasionally drink coffee and feel that caffeine aggravates your symptoms.
- Whenever the doctor suggests the management plan, you must ask if you would require surgery again and what is the success rate of repeat surgery?

Prompt Questions

- Doctor, why am I experiencing these symptoms again?
- Does this mean my surgery has failed?
- Why has my surgery failed?
- What needs to be done now?

EXAMINER'S INSTRUCTIONS AND STRUCTURED MARK SHEET

The examiner will mark the candidate on the basis of various tasks which are allotted to the candidate. Out of a total score of 20, the examiner can award a maximum of 18 marks, which are distributed between various candidate tasks as shown next. The role-player can award a maximum of 2 marks to the candidate. Each candidate task must be globally scored by the examiner.

Taking Relevant History from the Patient

- What is the patient's age?
- Obtain previous surgery records for obtaining information related to the type of surgery performed.
- History related to present symptoms of incontinence to characterise the type of incontinence:
  - *Stress incontinence*: Is incontinence present all the time or is aggravated by certain factors, e.g. coughing, sneezing, laughing, etc.?

- – *Urge incontinence*: Does she feel an urgent requirement to empty her bladder?
  - – *Mixed incontinence*: Whether symptoms related to both types of incontinence, i.e. stress incontinence and urge incontinence, are present?
- History related to basic urinary symptoms—urinary frequency, nocturia, and dysuria:
  - – *History of burning micturition or pain at the time of micturition*: The presence of dysuria will suggest an associated urinary tract infection (UTI). In the presence of these symptoms, the urinary symptoms may become worse and response to surgical treatment may not be as successful.
  - – Increased urinary frequency and nocturia could be indicative of underlying diabetes.
- *Symptoms of prolapse*: Dragging sensation in the vagina, feeling of incompletely emptying the bladder or rectum.
- *History of chronic cough and/or constipation*: Presence of both these conditions may affect the results of surgery.
- Basic gynaecological history including age of attaining menopause, smear history, and whether still sexually active.
- Obstetric history, previous deliveries, and size of babies.
- Fluid intake, especially quantity and timing of tea/coffee (i.e. caffeine intake).
- Family and social history, including history of smoking or intake of alcohol.

Marking Scheme

0	1	2	3	4	5	6
Fail		Borderline		Pass		

Investigations Required

Following the history, a general and pelvic examination must be undertaken. The presence of any abdominal masses or chest signs must be respectively ruled out on the abdominal and respiratory examination. A per speculum examination helps in ruling out atrophy of the genital tract, associated urethrocele, cystocele, uterine prolapse (if the patient has not had a hysterectomy), and an enterocele and a rectocele. It will also help in assessing the mobility around the urethra as she may require surgery. A bimanual pelvic examination may help in identifying any pelvic masses that could not be identified on abdominal examination.

In the examination, the candidate may be provided with the clinical findings or the results, which they may need to interpret. In case the findings of general and pelvic examination are not mentioned with the candidate's instruction, they can ask the examiner for the same. If the findings are available, the examiner would provide them to the candidate. Else, they would tell them that the findings are within normal limits.

Various investigations required in this case include the following:

- *Midstream specimen of urine*: This may be required to exclude the presence of UTIs. Presence of UTI may worsen the symptoms of incontinence.
- *Fasting blood glucose levels*: This may help rule out diabetes mellitus which may be associated with increased urinary frequency and nocturia.
- *Urine frequency and volume chart*: This may help provide additional information regarding the possible causes of patient's incontinence.
- *Urodynamic studies*: This may be required to help confirm the type of incontinence. The procedure is performed by inserting a catheter in the bladder and transducer in the rectum. The bladder is filled and the voiding pattern is observed. Though the procedure may not appear dignified, but it is not painful.
- Other investigations (e.g. urea and electrolytes, chest X-ray, and ECG) may be required as part of the preoperative assessment.

Marking Scheme

0	1	2	3	4	5	6
Fail		Borderline		Pass		

Devising a Subsequent Management Plan

- This patient has recurrent incontinence. Patient became symptomless post-surgery. Failure of previous treatment must be recognised in her management plan.
- Treatment depends on the cause of incontinence: stress incontinence, urge incontinence or mixed incontinence.
    - *Conservative therapy*: Pelvic floor exercise or physiotherapy
    - *Drugs for detrusor overactivity*: This could include drugs such as anticholinergic drugs, e.g. tolterodine (Detrusitol®), oxybutynin, etc.
    - *Surgery*: For repeat colposuspension, she needs to be referred to urogynaecologist.
        - Transvaginal tape or a sling procedure can be considered.
    - *Collagen implants*: This can be considered in case of a low compliance bladder. The success rates have not been found to be very high.
- Discussion of the complications related to the repeat procedure prior to the surgery.

Marking Scheme

0	1	2	3	4	5	6
Fail		Borderline		Pass		

Role-player's Score

The role-player can award a maximum of 2 marks to the candidate.

Marking Scheme

0	1	2
Role-player never wants to see candidate again	Role-player prepared to see candidate again	Role-player happy to see candidate again

Total score: /20

DISCUSSION

Issues

The treatment in this case depends upon the findings on history and physical examination and the results of the urodynamic investigations. In case of stress incontinence, surgical management, e.g. colposuspension or transvaginal taping (sling procedure) may be required.[10] This must be preferably performed by an urogynaecologist.

In the given case scenario, since the patient is experiencing recurrence of symptoms following surgery, a repeat surgery may be required. It is important to discuss the complications related to the repeat procedure with the patient prior to the surgery. It must be emphasised to the patient that the repeat surgery may be associated with a poorer success rate in comparison to that after a primary procedure. The patient usually needs to be followed-up for at least 5 years because there may be a recurrence rate of up to 60% after 5 years, following repeat surgery.

In case the patient is diagnosed to be suffering from urge incontinence or incontinence related to detrusor overactivity, the treatment of choice comprises of using anticholinergic drugs, e.g. tolterodine (Detrusitol®) or oxybutynin, or calcium channel blockers. In case of mixed incontinence, both surgery and medical treatment may be followed.[11] In case a low compliance bladder is diagnosed, treatment comprises of using collagen implants, bladder distension, and clamp cystoplasty. These procedures, however, are not associated with high rate of success for the treatment of this type of incontinence.

Pitfalls

Some common mistakes, which the candidates may commit, include offering the patient surgery for prolapse without confirming its presence or assuming that she has already had a hysterectomy. Another important mistake could be failing to justify or giving her the reason for any step taken in her management plan.

Variations

There could be a station, where the patient presents with first time incontinence. The type of incontinence may vary. The history may be suggestive of stress incontinence, urge incontinence or mixed incontinence (both stress and urge incontinence). Moreover, there may be small variations in the same scenario with a previous failed surgery, e.g. the women may give history of diabetes in which case there is a need to medically manage her diabetes first. In case she gives a history of UTIs, antibiotics need to be prescribed. If the patient has increased body mass index (BMI), she should be advised to lose weight loss. She should be advised physiotherapy and pelvic floor exercises in cases of mild prolapse. With such therapy, nearly 60% of cases are likely to notice improvement. The patient may benefit from hormone replacement therapy (HRT) if the vaginal tissues appear atrophic. In case she gives a history of increased fluid intake, especially caffeine, she must be advised to limit the fluid intake, especially in late evening or night to reduce nocturia.

OSCE STATION 3: POST-OPERATIVE MANAGEMENT OF THE PATIENT AFTER HYSTERECTOMY

Candidate's Instructions

Mary Grant, a 46-year-old woman, is scheduled for a hysterectomy and bilateral salpingo-oophorectomy. She is protein S deficient. You are about to meet the examiner who would ask you some questions pertaining to the management of this patient. The task is for 12 minutes (inclusive of 2 minutes of reading time). You have 10 minutes during which you should answer the examiner's questions. Examiner shall also test the core clinical skills domains covered in this station which are discussed next.

Core Clinical Skills Domains

Core clinical skills domains tested:

- Patient safety
- Communication with patients
- Communication with colleagues
- Information gathering
- Application of knowledge.

Module Tested

The module tested in this station is Module 3 or 'Post-operative Care'.

EXAMINER'S INSTRUCTIONS AND STRUCTURED MARK SHEET

The examiner will mark the candidate on the basis of various tasks which are allotted to the candidate. Out of a total score of 20, the examiner can award a maximum of 20 marks, which are distributed between various candidate tasks as shown next. Each candidate task must be globally scored by the examiner.

Examiner's Instructions

Familiarise yourself with the candidate's instructions and then ask the following four questions as written in candidate's task.

Co-ordination with Other Personnel

The candidate needs to co-ordinate with the following other personnel:
- On-duty consultant
- Anaesthetist
- Haematologist
- The candidate also needs to co-ordinate with the patient's partner to warn him about the seriousness of surgery.

Marking Scheme

0	1	2	3
Fail	Borderline		Pass

Justification of the Preoperative Management

- Due to the presence of thrombophilia, the patient is at an increased risk of VTE. Therefore, steps must be taken to reduce her risk for development of VTE perioperatively as well as during the post-operative period.
- The patient must be counselled regarding the various risks of thrombophilia, especially VTE. She must also be educated regarding the warning signs of VTE.
- From the beginning of her preoperative care, a haematologist should be involved in her perioperative care.
- Advice related to the use of most effective thromboprophylaxis in the form of heparin or low-molecular-weight heparin must be provided before surgery. If the patient has been taking warfarin, she needs to be switched to heparin before surgery is undertaken, preferably 1 day prior to surgery.
- Preoperatively, risk factors for deep vein thrombosis (DVT) (e.g. obesity, smoking, and concurrent infections) need to be identified. Efforts must be made to modify these risk factors.
- Pneumatic and thromboembolic deterrent (TED) stockings must be used.

Marking Scheme

0	1	2	3	4	5	6
Fail		Borderline		Pass		

Intraoperative Management

- Similar to the preoperative period, use of pneumatic and TED stockings should be continued during the intraoperative period.

- The duration of surgery must be kept to a minimum.
- Blood loss during surgery must be carefully controlled.
- Adequate hydration must also be maintained at the time of surgery.
- Thromboprophylaxis with heparin/Fragmin®/tinzaparin must be continued throughout the duration of surgery.

Marking Scheme

0	1	2	3	4	5
Fail		Borderline		Pass	

Post-operative Measures

- Maintenance of adequate hydration in the post-operative period is essential.
- The patient needs to be monitored regarding the warning signs of DVT or pulmonary embolism.
- Early mobilisation should be encouraged during the post-operative period.
- Thromboprophylaxis with heparin/Fragmin®/tinzaparin which had been initiated perioperatively should be continued for at least 5 days after surgery.
- Pneumatic/TED stockings must be continued during the post-operative period.
- Prophylactic antibiotics must be prescribed to reduce the risk of post-operative infection.
- Effort must be made towards early identification and treatment of complications such as infections (chest, wound, urinary tract, etc.) and thereby associated morbidity and immobility.
- Since the patient is only 46 years old and her ovaries have been removed during surgery, the requirement of HRT needs to be discussed with the patient. Before initiating HRT, benefits versus side-effects must be discussed with the patient.

Marking Scheme

0	1	2	3	4	5	6
Fail		Borderline		Pass		

Total score: /20

DISCUSSION

Issues

In this case, the most important aspect of management is the prevention of VTE in the preoperative, intraoperative, and post-operative periods. Thrombo-prophylaxis forms an important aspect of management. In some cases, the patient might have already been taking warfarin before surgery. In these cases, the oral thromboprophylaxis should be converted to a parenteral form before surgery. This shift should preferably be done a day prior to surgery.[12]

Another important aspect of the management of this patient involves the use of HRT. Since the patient is only 46 years old and would be undergoing hysterectomy along with oophorectomy, HRT in form of oestrogens needs to be prescribed. An important aspect of this station is that candidate must tell the examiner that they shall discuss the risks and the benefits of HRT with the patient before initiating it.

Pitfalls

The most common mistake committed by the candidates in this case is discussing the alternatives to surgery in this patient rather than the prevention of VTE. Not discussing the use of HRT in this patient is another flaw, which the candidates sometimes commit.

Variations

Variations in such stations could include discussion pertaining to other likely post-operative complications.

OSCE STATION 4: DAMAGE TO THE URETER AT THE TIME OF SURGERY

Candidate's Instructions

During an abdominal hysterectomy, you suspect that the ureter has been damaged on the right side. This is a structured viva where the examiner shall ask you some questions regarding the further course of management in this case. The task is for 12 minutes (inclusive of 2 minutes of reading time). You have 10 minutes during which you should answer the examiner's questions. Examiner shall also test the core clinical skills domains covered in this station which are discussed next.

Core Clinical Skills Domains

Core clinical skills domains tested:
- Patient safety
- Communication with patients
- Communication with colleagues
- Information gathering
- Application of knowledge.

Module Tested

The modules tested in this station are Module 2 or 'Core Surgical Skills' and Module 3 or 'Post-operative Care'.

EXAMINER'S INSTRUCTIONS AND STRUCTURED MARK SHEET

The examiner will mark the candidate on the basis of various tasks which are allotted to the candidate. Out of a total score of 20, the examiner can award a maximum of 20 marks, which are distributed between various candidate tasks as shown next. Each candidate task must be globally scored by the examiner.

Examiner's Instructions

Familiarise yourself with the candidate's instructions and then ask the following four questions:

> **Candidate's tasks:**
> - Which patients are likely to be an increased risk of injury to the urinary tract?
> - Outline the intraoperative steps you will take in theatre
> - Outline the post-operative steps
> - Enumerate steps for prevention of bladder injuries.

Patients Likely to be an Increased Risk of Injury to the Urinary Tract

- Patients with underlying pelvic or abdominal adhesions as a result of infections and endometriosis, or due to previous pelvic or abdominal surgeries (e.g. caesarean section, appendectomy, etc.).
- Patients with pelvic malignancy, undergoing surgery (e.g. Wertheim's hysterectomy in patients with cervical cancer).
- Patients with large abdominopelvic masses (e.g. large uterine fibroids or large ovarian tumours) undergoing surgery.
- *Patients undergoing vaginal hysterectomy*: Such patients may be at an increased risk of bladder injury at the time of peritoneal closure, buttressing of the bladder base, and dissection of bladder from the uterus. There may be at an increased risk of ureteric injury at the time of clamping the uterine artery.
- *Patients undergoing abdominal hysterectomy*: Such patients may be at an increased risk of ureteric injury at the time of clamping the uterine artery. There is also an increased risk of injury of bladder while dissection of bladder from the uterus.
- *Patients undergoing laparoscopy*: Visceral injury can occur at the time of insertion of Veress needle or the laparoscopic trocar using a wrong insertion technique.

Marking Scheme

0	1	2	3
Fail	Borderline		Pass

Intraoperative Steps to be Taken

- Maintaining a high index of suspicion especially in patients who are at an increased risk of such injury.

- Calling senior gynaecologist or urologist for help.
- Identification of the contralateral ureter (on the left side if there is an injury on the right side) to ensure that this is present. In case the ureter on contralateral side is absent, great care must be exercised during the repair of the damaged side.
- The surgeon needs to confirm if the injury or damage has actually occurred. The surgeon must try to trace the ureter and identify site of possible injury or damage (Fig. 4.3). The site of injury can be confirmed by observing urine flooding in the operative field. However, this may not always be easy.
- Additional measures may be taken to confirm the diagnosis. These include retrograde catheterisation of the ureter, retrograde cystourethroscopy, dye injection, and intraoperative intravenous urogram (IVU). For example, filling the bladder with methylene blue before dissecting the paraurethral tissues away from the proximal urethra and neck of the bladder during surgeries of bladder neck (e.g. colposuspension) and vagina is likely to help in early identification of any injuries.
- *Management of ureteric injury*: Once the ureteric injury is confirmed, various procedures can be undertaken to repair the injury. The various repair procedures which can be undertaken depending upon the type of injury include end-to-end anastomosis; splint with ureteric catheter; psoas hitch (Figs. 4.4A to C); raising a Boari flap (Figs. 4.5A to C); reimplantation of the ureters into the bladder; ileal conduit; etc. If possible, immediate end-to-end anastomosis appears to be the ideal procedure in case of ureteric injury. Additionally, a ureteric stent may be important to splint the site of anastomosis. In some cases, it may be possible to raise a Boari flap. This procedure helps in ensuring that the ureter remains functional and reduces the chances of harm to the kidneys. In most of these cases, a urologist requires to be called in order to perform these surgeries.

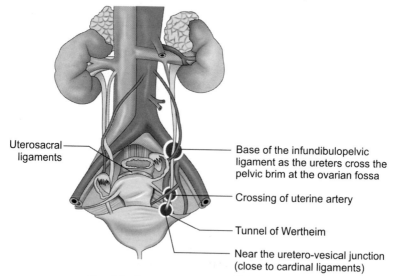

Uterosacral ligaments

Base of the infundibulopelvic ligament as the ureters cross the pelvic brim at the ovarian fossa

Crossing of uterine artery

Tunnel of Wertheim

Near the uretero-vesical junction (close to cardinal ligaments)

Fig. 4.3: Common sites of ureteric injuries.

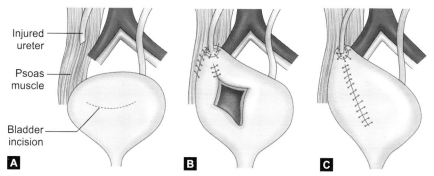

Figs. 4.4A to C: Psoas hitch. (A) The bladder is incised transversely and mobilised to reach the shortened ureter to achieve a tension-free anastomosis; (B) The bladder is fixed to the psoas muscle, and (C) The incision is repaired in a vertical manner which allows 'elongation' of the bladder.

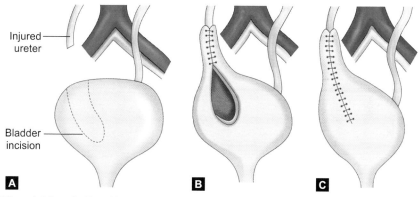

Figs. 4.5A to C: Boari flap. (A) A wide-based flap is developed by an anterior bladder wall incision; (B) The flap is brought towards the ureter to achieve a tension-free anastomosis, and (C) The bladder incision is closed in a tubular manner to allow up to 12–15 cm of additional length.

- In case, the injury is non-crushing type or the ureter was transfixed, simply removing the stitch and stenting it, may be sufficient. On the other hand, if the injury is crushing type and the crushed segment is likely to be necrotic, it is better to excise it and undertake end-to-end anastomosis.

Marking Scheme

0	1	2	3	4	5
Fail		Borderline		Pass	

Post-operative Management

- Administration of prophylactic antibiotics.
- The patient must be monitored for symptoms and signs of ureteric injury (Box 4.1) and early warning signs of urinary peritonitis (abdominal

> **BOX 4.1:** Symptoms and signs of ureteric injury.
>
> - Fever
> - Haematuria
> - Flank pain
> - Abdominal distension
> - Abscess formation or sepsis
> - Peritonitis or ileus
> - Urinary leakage (vaginally or via abdominal wound)
> - Secondary hypertension
> - Retroperitoneal urinoma
> - Post-operative anuria

tenderness, distension, fever, fluid in the abdomen, oliguria, difficulty in passing gas or having bowel movement, etc.)
- She should be counselled about the injury and the course of management which would be followed.
- An incident form should be completed for risk-management purposes.
- Once the healing is thought to be complete, the ureteric stent should be removed.
- The patient may be then offered an IVU to confirm the patency of the ureter and a functioning kidney.
- The patient must be followed-up to ensure that no future complications occur.

Marking Scheme

0	1	2	3	4	5	6
Fail		Borderline		Pass		

Steps for Prevention of Bladder Injuries

- Recognition of those patients who may be at a risk of such injuries.
- The most important single step to take in case of abdominal and laparoscopic surgeries is to empty the bladder prior to surgery.
- Some surgeons advocate the use of suprapubic drainage with a needle to help reduce the risk of UTIs associated with urinary catheterisation.
- Meticulous and systematic surgical technique to be followed.
- Early recognition and management of such complications when they occur.
- If the surgeon feels that he/she lacks the expertise to deal with them, they must summon senior help.
- During laparoscopy, it is important to direct the Veress needle and the trocar towards the pelvis but away from the bladder.
- If pelvic or abdominal adhesions are suspected, the surgeon must adopt a more superior approach while entering the abdominal cavity in order to bypass an adherent bladder.
- Blunt dissection is likely to be safer than sharp dissection at the time of surgery.

- If there is any bleeding around the bladder base, this must be clearly identified before securing haemostasis.
- Blind diathermy or suturing must be avoided as it may result in injuries to the bladder.
- The surgeon should have a detailed understanding regarding the anatomy of pelvis. An understanding regarding the relationship of the bladder to the uterus and the anterior abdominal wall is important for minimising the risk of injury to the bladder and/or the ureters.
- Early recognition and correction of injuries when they occur.
- Once an injury is suspected, it must be confirmed. This could be done by filling the bladder with a dye, such as methylene blue. Flooding of the operative site with clear fluid is also likely to raise the suspicion of bladder or ureteric injury.
- Occurrence of haematuria or urinary incontinence in the post-operative period could be indicative of potential injury to the bladder. These complications must be investigated and early treatment must be offered to prevent further damage.

Marking Scheme

0	1	2	3	4	5	6
Fail		Borderline		Pass		

Total score: /20

DISCUSSION

Issues

Though the ureteric or bladder injuries may be sometimes difficult to recognise, such injuries can commonly occur in difficult gynaecological cases as well as difficult obstetric surgeries. Bladder injuries are most likely to occur either during introduction of the laparoscopic port or dissection of the bladder away from the uterus (in abdominal and vaginal hysterectomy), separation of bladder from adhesions, during a colposuspension or anterior repair, etc. Therefore, a high index of suspicion must be maintained by the surgeon at the time of these surgeries to rule out the injuries of urinary tract.

A candidate at ST5 level must be competent enough to deal with such complications. An ST5 candidate must also be competent enough to take steps for prevention of ureteric injuries (Box 4.2). Though at this level, the candidate is not expected to perform the repair of ureteric injuries, they must be competent enough to recognise such injury, call for senior help (e.g. gynaecologist consultant, urologist) and outline the management plan.

Pitfalls

The candidate must carefully read the tasks they are supposed to perform. An important mistake committed by the candidate at this stage could be discussion

> **BOX 4.2:** Steps for prevention of ureteric injuries at the time of surgery.
>
> - Adequate exposure
> - Avoid blind clamping of blood vessels
> - Ureteric dissection and direct visualisation
> - Mobilisation of the bladder away from operative site
> - Using short diathermy applications

pertaining to the prevention of ureteric injury rather the management of ureteric or bladder injuries, when the examiner wants to know about the management of such injuries. Discussion of steps for minimising bowel injury during gynaecological surgery (without being asked about) is another mistake which the candidate may commit.

Variations

The various variations, which could be introduced in this station, include the injuries occurring at the time of laparoscopic or hysteroscopic surgeries in addition to laparotomy. Besides the occurrence of injury to the urinary tract, the candidate may be asked about dealing with other surgery-related complications, e.g. dealing with bowel injury or difficulties encountered at the various stages of the surgery (for example modifications of surgical incisions due to the difficulty encountered while entering the abdomen).

OSCE STATION 5: PREOPERATIVE ASSESSMENT OF PATIENTS PRIOR TO SURGERY

Candidate's Instructions

You are the registrar responsible for today's operating list. Your consultant would be in the hospital but has an important meeting and would prefer not to be disturbed. You now have to take the preoperative ward round. You are about to meet the examiner. Examiner will ask you some questions about what you would normally do with each patient preoperatively, including the counselling you shall be offering them. The task is for 12 minutes (inclusive of 2 minutes of reading time). You have 10 minutes during which you should answer the examiner's questions. Examiner shall also test the core clinical skills domains covered in this station which are discussed next.

1. Mrs Jacqueline Andrews, a 29-year-old woman, listed for a laparoscopically assisted vaginal hysterectomy for heavy periods that failed to respond to medical treatment.
2. Mrs Hester Greene, a 60-year-old woman with hesitance, frequency and stress urinary incontinence, listed for a cystoscopy.
3. Mrs Jodie Revell, A 26-year-old nulliparous woman, listed for a diagnostic laparoscopy for deep dyspareunia and dysmenorrhoea.

Core Clinical Skills Domains

Core clinical skills domains tested:
- Patient safety
- Communication with patients
- Information gathering
- Application of knowledge.

Module Tested

The module tested in this station is Module 2 or 'Core Surgical Skills'.

EXAMINER'S INSTRUCTIONS AND STRUCTURED MARK SHEET

Each of the cases should be answered according to the structure described next. Each case must be answered separately and not as a universal process. Each case should be marked as determined from the reckoner. Total global score should be out of 40 marks but the overall score for the station should be out of 20 marks by dividing the global score by 2. Please ask the candidate the following questions as they are written. Do not prompt and do not award half marks.

1. Mrs Jacqueline Andrews, a 29-year-old woman, is listed for a laparoscopically assisted vaginal hysterectomy for heavy periods that failed to respond to medical treatment.

Q. What relevant history you would want to know?
- Ask her about her main symptoms to make sure that they have not changed since the time of her first presentation
- Confirm that she knows that she is scheduled for laparoscopically assisted vaginal hysterectomy
- Does the patient understand what the surgery involves?
- History of any previous surgery, especially abdominal or pelvic
- Was the option of Mirena insertion discussed with her?
- Has the option of endometrial ablation being discussed?
- Has the option of subtotal hysterectomy been discussed?
- When was her last menstrual period?
- Has the pregnancy test been done?

Marking Scheme

0	1	2	3	4
Fail	Borderline		Pass	

Q. Investigations you would want to be done?
- Findings on ultrasonography
- Any available results of endometrial histology

- Full blood count (FBC)
- Pregnancy test
- Cervical smear.

Marking Scheme

0	1	2	3	4
Fail	Borderline		Pass	

Q. Other aspects of the procedure you would like to know?
- Does she understand what operation she is having?
- Confirm whether conservation of the ovaries has been discussed.
- Has the patient been counselled about the risks of complications, especially those associated with laparoscopic surgery.
- Has the need for thromboprophylaxis in the post-operative period been discussed?

Marking Scheme

0	1	2	3
Fail	Borderline		Pass

Q. What complications can occur in the post-operative period, which you must tell her about?
She should be warned about the following complications of surgery:
- Haemorrhage
- Injury to viscera (e.g. bowel, bladder, ureter, etc.)
- Complications of anaesthesia and laparoscopic surgery
- Other complications (e.g. infection, urinary complications) and their management
- Recovery, including stay in hospital and time off work
- Insertion of an intravenous (IV) line (tube inserted in the arm to supply IV fluids) and urinary catheter (tube to drain the urinary bladder).

Marking Scheme

0	1	2	3
Fail	Borderline		Pass

Q. Anything else you want to consider before checking her consent form?
- Examine her abdomen to rule out the presence of any abdominal mass
- Does she want to ask any other questions?

Marking Scheme

0	1	2
Fail	Borderline	Pass

2. Mrs Hester Greene, a 60-year-old woman with hesitance, frequency and stress urinary incontinence, is listed for a cystoscopy.

Q. Relevant history you would want to know?
- Kind of incontinence (stress or urge)?
- History suggestive of urinary infection (e.g. dysuria, abdominal pain, fever, etc.)
- Past obstetrics and gynaecology history
- Past history of any surgery.

Marking Scheme

0	1	2	3	4
Fail	Borderline		Pass	

Q. Investigations you would want to be done?
- FBC
- Urine routine microscopy
- Urine culture sensitivity.

Marking Scheme

0	1	2
Fail	Borderline	Pass

Q. Other aspects of the procedure you would like to know?
- The patient must be asked if she understands the procedure she would be going through?
- Has she been counselled about the complications associated with cystoscopy?
- Though the procedure is done under anaesthesia, the patient may feel pain and discomfort while cystoscope is inserted inside the urethra into the bladder.

Marking Scheme

0	1	2
Fail	Borderline	Pass

Q. What would you warn her post-operatively?
- Minor complications can occur in the post-operative period. These include the following:
  - *Infection*: Infection may rarely occur. Risks for developing an infection are lowered with administration of an antibiotic prior to and after the procedure.
  - *Bleeding*: Bleeding in urine may sometimes occur. Serious bleeding rarely occurs.

- – *Pain*: Abdominal pain and/or burning sensation at the time of passing urine can sometimes occur.
- – *Urinary problems*: There may be difficulty in passing urine, urinary retention or sometimes even urinary incontinence.
- She must be told about the recovery period and the duration of hospital stay.

Marking Scheme

0	1	2
Fail	Borderline	Pass

Q. Anything else you want to consider before checking her consent form?
- Does she want to ask any other question?
- Usually no relation with the menstrual cycles, therefore no need to ask about the LMP.

Marking Scheme

0	1	2
Fail	Borderline	Pass

3. Mrs Jodie Revell, A 26-year-old nulliparous woman, is listed for a diagnostic laparoscopy for deep dyspareunia and dysmenorrhoea.

Q. What relevant history would you want to know?
- Nature of pain (dull or throbbing or spasmodic)
- Since how long she has been experiencing pain
- Relationship of pain with menstrual cycles
- Exact site of pain
- Previous obstetrics and gynaecology history
- Past history of any surgery (especially abdominal or pelvic).

Marking Scheme

0	1	2	3	4
Fail	Borderline		Pass	

Q. Investigations you would want to be done?
- Ultrasound findings
- FBC
- Pregnancy test
- Cervical smear.

Marking Scheme

0	1	2
Fail	Borderline	Pass

Classic gun-metal, blue-gray spots	'Raspberry' spots with shaggy tissue	Flat or raised white tissue, like scarring	Clear 'berries' with small peaks	Chocolate cysts filled with old blood

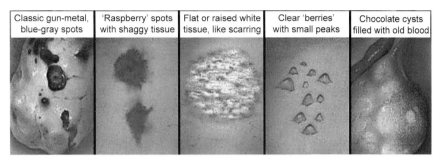

Fig. 4.6: Various lesions of endometriosis.

Q. Other aspects of the procedure you would like to know?
- Does she know what kind of surgery would be done on her?
- In case diagnosis of endometriosis is made on laparoscopy (Fig. 4.6), diathermy or excision of the endometriotic lesions would be useful and may be performed.

Marking Scheme

0	1	2
Fail	Borderline	Pass

Q. What would you warn her post-operatively?
- Injury to bowel or bladder or ureter, etc.
- Number of skin incisions, their approximate size and position.

Marking Scheme

0	1	2
Fail	Borderline	Pass

Q. Anything else you want to consider before checking her consent form?
- Her abdomen needs to be examined
- When was her LMP?
- Ask her if she has any questions regarding the procedure.

Marking Scheme

0	1	2
Fail	Borderline	Pass

Total score: /40 = score/2 = /20

DISCUSSION

Issues

At such kinds of station, the candidate is expected to demonstrate their competency in undertaking a preoperative ward round. Such kinds of stations are usually high scoring. Therefore, the candidate must try to give all the answers within the stipulated time of 10 minutes.

Pitfalls

The major mistake in such kinds of stations is that if the candidates fumble on a particular question, they mess up all the following questions. However, they must remember that even if they get stuck up on a particular question, they must go on to answer the next question because each question is scored individually based on the reckoner described previously in the text.

Variations

Such kind of station is similar to a day on the preoperative ward, where the doctor has to counsel the patients who are posted in the list for surgery. In such kind of stations, there can be a wide variety of patients posted for surgeries in both obstetrics and gynaecology similar to a preoperative ward.

OSCE STATION 6: PRIORITISATION ON LABOUR WARD

Candidate's Instructions

You are the registrar on call for the labour ward. You have been given a handover at 08:30 am as you arrived in the hospital for the morning shift. The sister-in-charge quickly runs through the problems giving you a brief résumé of the 10 women on the delivery suite on board (also attached below). She tells you that it is busy and she is short of staff. There are six midwives (DB, CD, BB, ST, MM, and TT) on duty. DB is in charge co-ordinator. DB, CD, and ST are capable of inserting a Venflon®, DB and BB are able to suture episiotomies, whereas MM and TT are newly qualified midwives. On duty with you are an ST1 in her twelfth month of career training and a third-year specialist ST3.

You shall next meet the examiner who shall discuss with you your decisions and your justifications for making those decisions.

The task is for 12 minutes (inclusive of 2 minutes of reading time). The candidate has 10 minutes to explain the following:

Candidate's tasks:
- The tasks that need to be done on the delivery suite
- Their order of priority in which the patients should be seen and managed
- The staff he/she would allocate to each patient.

Patient Information

The 10 patients are as follows:

Room 1: A 27-year-old, para 1 woman with 39 weeks of gestation, undiagnosed breech presentation, having uterine contractions since last 12 hours, just admitted in the labour ward. On vaginal examination (VE), cervix is effaced and 5 cm dilated.

Room 2: Mrs MT, a primigravida at 35 weeks' gestation with premature rupture of foetal membranes and having variable decelerations.

Room 3: Mrs Marsh with uncomplicated twins in early labour at 37 weeks' gestation.

Room 4: Mrs Andrews, a primipara who has been fully dilated and pushing for 2 hours.

Room 5: Mrs Khan, a para 6 patient is admitted at 39 completed weeks of gestation. She has been having regular uterine contractions and her membranes have ruptured spontaneously, with escape of clear fluid. She was fully effaced and 7 cm dilated at 7 am.

Room 6: Mrs PJ with abdominal pain at 26 weeks' gestation.

Room 7: Mrs Green, a 42-year-old primigravida at 38 weeks' gestation, presenting with spontaneous labour shows meconium-stained liquor. She is having good uterine contractions; CTG was observed to be suspicious. At 8 am, scalp blood pH was 7.23 and cervix was 8 cm dilated.

Room 8: Primigravida who delivered at 8 am and is awaiting repair of her episiotomy.

Room 9: Uncomplicated primigravida at 41 weeks in normal labour.

Room 10: Mrs Adams, para 3, previous 2 caesarean deliveries, intact membranes posted for elective caesarean section at 39 weeks of gestation.

The examiner will also test the core clinical skills domains covered in this station which are discussed next.

Core Clinical Skills Domains

Core clinical skills domains tested:
• Patient safety
• Communication with colleagues
• Information gathering
• Application of knowledge.

Module Tested

The modules tested in this station are Module 6 or 'Management of Labour' and Module 7 or 'Management of Delivery.'

EXAMINER'S INSTRUCTIONS AND STRUCTURED MARK SHEET

The candidate is required to identify the task(s) that need to be done for each patient, the priority in which these patients should be seen and managed, and the member of staff who will be allocated to do these tasks.

The examiner must discuss each case briefly, and mark them globally. If there are 10 cases, then each must be scored out of 4, and the overall score must be divided by 2. If there are eight cases, then each must be scored out of 5, and the overall score be divided by 2.

The 10 patients discussed above are as follows:

Room 1: A 27-year-old, para 1 woman with 39 weeks of gestation, undiagnosed breech presentation, having uterine contractions since last 12 hours, just admitted in the labour ward. On VE, cervix is effaced and 5 cm dilated.

- *Tasks:* She must be assessed for suitability for a vaginal delivery. The options for delivery, whether by caesarean or vaginal route, must be discussed with the woman and her partner. The anaesthetist must be informed. An IV line needs to be inserted and blood needs to be taken for a FBC and group and save. If the decision for a caesarean delivery has been taken, the relevant consent needs to be taken. A repeat VE may be required to assess her progress of labour.
- *Priority:* Urgent review.
- *Personnel:* Registrar (ST3).

Marking Scheme

0	1	2	3	4
Fail	Borderline		Pass	

Room 2: Mrs MT, a primigravida at 35 weeks' gestation with premature rupture of foetal membranes and having variable decelerations.

- *Tasks:* Need to exclude cord prolapse or compression. A quick VE needs to be done in order to exclude cord prolapse. The patient must be turned on the side to see the effect on the foetal heart rate. If cardiotocography (CTG) becomes normal, the probable cause can be considered as cord compression. Nevertheless, the patient requires monitoring with CTG. The patient may require delivery in case there is deterioration in the CTG trace.
- *Priority:* Urgent review.
- *Personnel:* Registrar (ST1).

Marking Scheme

0	1	2	3	4
Fail	Borderline		Pass	

Room 3: Mrs Marsh with uncomplicated twins in early labour at 37 weeks' gestation.

- *Tasks:* An IV line needs to be inserted and blood needs to be taken for a FBC and group and save. Both the foetal heart rates must be assessed. Anaesthetist and paediatrician need to be notified.
- *Priority:* Semi-urgent.
- *Personnel:* Midwife CD.

Marking Scheme

0	1	2	3	4
Fail	Borderline		Pass	

Room 4: Mrs Andrews, a primipara who has been fully dilated and pushing for 2 hours.
- *Tasks*: There is a requirement to do a VE to evaluate the reasons for her failure to deliver (malposition or malpresentation or cephalopelvic disproportion). The foetal health also needs to be assessed by performing a CTG.
- *Priority*: Urgent.
- *Personnel*: Midwife DB.

Marking Scheme

0	1	2	3	4
Fail	Borderline		Pass	

Room 5: Mrs Khan, a para 6 patient, is admitted at 39 completed weeks of gestation. She has been having regular uterine contractions and her membranes have ruptured spontaneously, with escape of clear fluid. She was fully effaced and 7 cm dilated at 7 am.
- *Tasks*: The VE needs to be done to assess if she is fully dilated and must be allowed to deliver. She would require an IV line and active management of the third stage of labour because she is a grand multipara. Labour analgesia must be considered if she is in too much pain. In that case, the anaesthetist needs to be called. Foetal well-being needs to be assessed.
- *Priority*: Urgent.
- *Personnel*: Midwife ST.

Marking Scheme

0	1	2	3	4
Fail	Borderline		Pass	

Room 6: Mrs PJ with abdominal pain at 26 weeks' gestation.
- *Tasks*: Assess CTG, more information needs to be taken from the patient regarding nature of pain. Needs to assess if there is any associated bleeding or leaking per vaginum. Abruption placenta needs to be ruled out, especially if there is a history of bleeding.
- *Priority*: Semi-urgent.
- *Personnel*: Midwife MM.

Marking Scheme

0	1	2	3	4
Fail	Borderline		Pass	

Room 7: Mrs Green, a 42-year-old primigravida at 38 weeks' gestation, presenting with spontaneous labour shows meconium-stained liquor. She is having good uterine contractions; CTG was observed to be suspicious. At 8 am, scalp blood pH was 7.23 and cervix was 8 cm dilated.

Tasks: Needs repeat foetal blood sampling (FBS) in case she is not yet ready for the delivery. Whether delivery needs to be expedited using instrumental delivery or not, depends upon the results of foetal scalp pH and the foetal heart trace. Continuous CTG monitoring must be done.

- *Priority*: Urgent.
- *Personnel*: Registrar (self).

Marking Scheme

0	1	2	3	4
Fail	Borderline		Pass	

Room 8: Primigravida who delivered at 8 am and is awaiting repair of her episiotomy.

- *Tasks*: Needs suturing of episiotomy. A quick VE needs to be done to assess the state of cervix and presence of any tears or hematoma. Target for a labour ward is that repair of an episiotomy must be performed within an hour of delivery.
- *Priority*: Semi-urgent (in view of the timing of delivery).
- *Personnel*: Midwife BB.

Marking Scheme

0	1	2	3	4
Fail	Borderline		Pass	

Room 9: Uncomplicated primigravida at 41 weeks in normal labour.

- *Tasks*: Normal labouring patient. No action needs to be immediately taken, but the patient and the foetus both need to be monitored.
- *Priority*: No immediate action.
- *Personnel*: To be managed by midwife TT.

Marking Scheme

0	1	2	3	4
Fail	Borderline		Pass	

Room 10: Mrs Adams, para 3, previous 2 caesarean deliveries, intact membranes posted for an elective caesarean section at 39 weeks of gestation.

- *Tasks*: Check if the consent has been taken:
  - Blood sample needs to be taken for group and save
  - Results of the recent FBC and methicillin-resistant *Staphylococcus aureus* (MRSA) swab need to be checked
  - Assessment of prophylactic therapy for VTE
  - Check, what was the last time she ate and drank?
- *Priority*: Routine.
- *Personnel*: ST3 or self.

Marking Scheme

0	1	2	3	4
Fail	Borderline		Pass	

Total score: /40 = score/2 = /20

Priority of Tasks and Staff Allocation

Priorities for review are as follows: Room No. 7 is at the highest priority followed by rooms 1 and 2. It would be appropriate for the candidate to manage the Room No. 7 by himself/herself. ST3 can be in Room No. 1, while the ST1 can be in Room No. 2. Another patient who needs to be urgently managed is in Room No. 4 and must be managed by the midwife, DB. She probably can be helped by the candidate themselves or any other registrar as and when they get free. Midwife BB should suture the episiotomy in Room No. 8. This, however, is not an urgent task in lieu of the timing of delivery. After the urgent tasks have been sorted out, the medical staff depending upon their availability could review the other patients with semi-urgent or routine requirements.

DISCUSSION

Issues

These kinds of stations aim at testing the candidate's ability to prioritise the patients based on the level of urgency of their problems and safely manage the labour ward. The candidate needs to show a well thought-out and confident approach and be able to justify all their decisions. Since in this station, the consultant is away, the candidates must refrain themselves from saying that they would take their consultant's advice. Instead they must be able to demonstrate their ability to take control of the labour ward in absence of their consultant. Nevertheless, it would be wise for the candidate to mention that they shall call the consultant and inform him/her about their decisions. Sometimes, there may not be a single correct answer. However, if the candidates can sufficiently justify their decisions, they are likely to score well.

In such kind of stations, typically there will be 1–3 patients who would require an urgent review, 1–3 who can be left for a while, and the rest for whom the candidate would be required to take a decision and to justify it as well. The candidates need to prove to the examiner that they know what is important, that they follow a structured and organised approach and have the capability to handover the responsibility to other staff members. The candidate should give clear and concise answers.

Pitfalls

The candidates must remember that they would not be able to do everything on their own. They must try to delegate the less important tasks to the other members of the staff. Simultaneously, the candidates need to ensure that the staff would communicate with them in case of occurrence of any complications or problems. The candidate should not waste their time in reading out the details related to each patient because these details would also be available inside the station. For each patient, they should give a diagnosis along with a differential diagnosis, if required. They should also briefly explain the management plan.

Variations

The OSCE stations related to the prioritisation of patients include prioritisation of the patients in a labour ward or a delivery suite or prioritisation of the patients for an operative list in the preoperative ward or prioritisation of the patients referred by the GP.

OSCE STATION 7: PRIORITISATION OF THE PATIENTS FOR SURGERY

Candidate's Instructions

You are asked to go through a consultant's gynaecology waiting list. Your task is to review the list and prioritise the patients based on the level of urgency of their surgery. You would be required to classify the patients' surgery into routine (within 3 months), urgent (within 4 weeks), target (31/62-day cancer target rule), or emergency (immediate admission). The candidate would be required to perform the following tasks:

Candidate's tasks:

Advising the waiting list manager regarding the following:
- Appropriateness of the procedure
- Venue of proposed treatment (outpatient department, day unit or inpatient)
- Special needs (if any)
- Priority of assignment—routine (18 weeks from referral), urgent (within 4 weeks), target (31/62-day cancer target rule), or emergency (immediate admission).

The task is for 12 minutes (inclusive of 2 minutes of reading time). You have 10 minutes for this station. You shall be meeting the examiner to whom you shall be describing your actions and offering explanations wherever appropriate. You shall be awarded marks for your ability to manage and prioritise the cases.

Patient Information

The 10 patients are as follows:

Case 1: Mrs Ford, a 48-year-old severely asthmatic woman on Ventolin® and steroids with focal atypical endometrial hyperplasia, listed for hysterectomy along with bilateral salpingo-oophorectomy.

Case 2: Miss Mary, an 18-year-old girl who presented with severe dysmenorrhoea and heavy periods since past 1 year, listed for a diagnostic laparoscopy.

Case 3: Mrs Hammond, a 67-year-old woman with a painless ulcer on her right labium majorum, listed for an excisional biopsy.

Case 4: An 8-year-old girl, Susan Wilde, with a bloody vaginal discharge of 2 weeks' duration listed for examination under anaesthesia.

Case 5: Mrs Dunn, 38-year-old woman with a large pelvic mass, likely ovarian cyst, CA125 = 45 IU/mL, posted for staging laparotomy.

Case 6: Mrs Bryant, a 77-year-old widower living on her own, on the list for myomectomy for fibroid uterus and menorrhagia; her haemoglobin level is 8.0 g%.

Case 7: Mrs Adams, a 28-year-old woman with a diagnosis of primary infertility placed on the list for a diagnostic laparoscopy and dye test.

Case 8: Mrs Marsh, a 48-year-old diabetic woman, on the list for a Wertheim's hysterectomy for carcinoma of the cervix stage 1A.

Case 9: Mrs Andrews, an 80-year-old patient with procidentia and urinary incontinence. Treatment with pessary has failed in her. She is Jehovah's Witness and her preoperative haemoglobin level is 8 g%. She is posted for vaginal hysterectomy and pelvic floor repair.

Case 10: Ms Joan, 18-year-old woman, presented with a recent abnormal smear; cervical biopsy; cervical intraepithelial neoplasia 3. She is posted for the large loop excision of transformation zone (LLETZ).

The examiner shall also test the core clinical skills domains covered in this station which are discussed next.

Core Clinical Skills Domains

Core clinical skills domains tested:

- Patient safety
- Communication with patients
- Information gathering
- Application of knowledge.

Module Tested

The module tested in this station is Module 2 or 'Core Surgical Skills.'

EXAMINER'S INSTRUCTIONS AND STRUCTURED MARK SHEET

The examiner must discuss each case briefly, and mark them globally. If there are 10 cases, then each must be scored out of 4, and the overall score must be divided by 2. If there are eight cases, then each must be scored out of 5, and the overall score be divided by 2.

Case 1: Mrs Ford, a 48-year-old severely asthmatic woman on Ventolin® and steroids with focal atypical endometrial hyperplasia, listed for hysterectomy along with bilateral salpingo-oophorectomy.

Appropriateness: Appropriate.

Category: Urgent.

Venue: Inpatient.

Additional procedure: The surgery must preferably be performed by gynaecological oncologists. Physician review and lung function test must be done prior to the surgery in view of her asthma.

Marking Scheme

0	1	2	3	4
Fail	Borderline		Pass	

Case 2: Miss Mary, an 18-year-old girl who presented with severe dysmenorrhoea and heavy periods since past 1 year, listed for a diagnostic laparoscopy.

Appropriateness: Inappropriate.

Category: There is no requirement for surgical treatment in this case.

Venue: There is no requirement for surgical treatment in this case. She can be treated in the outpatient department.

Additional procedure: Medical treatment with combined oral contraceptive pills must be administered.

Marking Scheme

0	1	2	3	4
Fail	Borderline		Pass	

Case 3: Mrs Hammond, a 67-year-old woman with a painless ulcer on her right labium majorum, listed for an excisional biopsy.

Appropriateness: Appropriate.

Category: Urgent.

Venue: Inpatient.

Additional procedure: Surgery should preferably be performed by gynaecological oncologist.

Marking Scheme

0	1	2	3	4
Fail	Borderline		Pass	

Case 4: An 8-year-old girl, Susan Wilde, with a bloody vaginal discharge of 2 weeks' duration listed for examination under anaesthesia.

Appropriateness: Appropriate.

Category: Urgent.

Venue: Daycare.

Additional procedure: Ensure bed on paediatric ward, using local anaesthetic cream before insertion of a cannula (drip).

Marking Scheme

0	1	2	3	4
Fail	Borderline		Pass	

Case 5: Mrs Dunn, a 38-year-old woman with a large pelvic mass, likely ovarian cyst, CA125 = 45 IU/mL, posted for staging laparotomy.
Appropriateness: Appropriate.
Category: Target.
Venue: Inpatient.
Additional procedure: Management by a multidisciplinary team comprising of an gynaecological oncologist; consultant gynaecologist must be present; MRI.

Marking Scheme

0	1	2	3	4
Fail	Borderline		Pass	

Case 6: Mrs Bryant, a 77-year-old widower living on her own, on the list for myomectomy for fibroid uterus and menorrhagia; her haemoglobin level is 8.0 g%.
Appropriateness: Inappropriate. It would be more appropriate to consider total abdominal hysterectomy or subtotal hysterectomy in this case.
Category: Routine.
Venue: Inpatient.
Additional procedure: Correction of anaemia prior to surgery using oral iron therapy. Hormonal suppression with gonadotropin-releasing hormone analogues can also be tried. Social support must be arranged after surgery.

Marking Scheme

0	1	2	3	4
Fail	Borderline		Pass	

Case 7: Mrs Adams, a 28-year-old woman with a diagnosis of primary infertility placed on the list for a diagnostic laparoscopy and dye test.
Appropriateness: Appropriate.
Category: Routine.
Venue: Daycare.
Additional procedures: Semen analysis and 21-day progesterone levels need to be done. Pregnancy test on the day of surgery also requires to be done.

Marking Scheme

0	1	2	3	4
Fail	Borderline		Pass	

Case 8: Mrs Marsh, a 48-year-old diabetic woman, on the list for a Wertheim's hysterectomy for carcinoma of the cervix stage 1A.

Appropriateness: Appropriate.

Category: Urgent, she should be first on the list (being a diabetic patient).

Venue: Inpatient.

Additional procedure: Sliding scale insulin therapy must be administered.

Marking Scheme

0	1	2	3	4
Fail	Borderline		Pass	

Case 9: Mrs Andrews, an 80-year-old patient with procidentia and urinary incontinence. Treatment with pessary has failed in her. She is Jehovah's Witness and her preoperative haemoglobin level is 8 g%. She is posted for vaginal hysterectomy and pelvic floor repair.

Appropriateness: Appropriate.

Category: Routine.

Venue: Inpatient.

Additional procedure: Haemoglobin levels must be built prior to surgery (preferably using oral iron therapy). The candidate should also discuss with the patient the preoperative treatment of anaemia and the requirement of a normal blood count before surgery. Consent must be taken using the special operation form prior to the surgery (in view of the patient being a Jehovah's Witness).

Marking Scheme

0	1	2	3	4
Fail	Borderline		Pass	

Case 10: Ms Joan, 18-year-old woman, presented with a recent abnormal smear, cervical biopsy, and cervical intraepithelial neoplasia 3. She is posted for LLETZ.

Appropriateness: Appropriate.

Category: Urgent.

Venue: Daycare.

Additional procedures: Treatment must be instituted within the target of NHSCSP guidelines (National Health Services Cervical Screening Programme).

Marking Scheme

0	1	2	3	4
Fail	Borderline		Pass	

Total score: $/40 = $ score$/2 = /20$

DISCUSSION

Issues

Similar to the previous station, this station also tests the candidate's ability to prioritise the patients for surgery on the basis of their urgency. The answers are not clear-cut and sometimes there may be no correct answer. The candidate must, therefore, follow a common sense approach.

Pitfalls

The candidates must not make an effort to memorise the particulars of each patient during the 2 minutes of their reading time, while they are outside the examination booth. Rather they must focus on the management aspects of each patient. Details related to the various patients would also be provided inside the examination booth.

Variations

As previously mentioned, the OSCE stations related to the prioritisation of patients include prioritisation of the patients in a labour ward or a delivery suite or prioritisation of the patients for an operative list in the preoperative ward or prioritisation of the patients referred by the GP.

REFERENCES

1. Aspden P, Corrigan J, Wolcott J, et al. (Eds). Patient safety: Achieving a New Standard for Care. Washington, DC: National Academies Press; 2004.
2. Palmieri PA, DeLucia PR, Ott TE, et al. The anatomy and physiology of error in adverse health care events. Advances in Health Care Management. 2008;7:33-68.
3. Patients Association. (2013). Good practice standards for NHS Complaints Handling. [online] Available from https://www.patients-association.org.uk/wp-content/uploads/2014/06/Good-Practice-standards-for-NHS-Complaints-HandlingSept-2013.pdf [Accessed December 2017].
4. Cancer Waiting Times Team. Cancer Waiting Times: A Guide (Version 9.0). Leeds: Cancer Waiting Times Team; 2015.
5. Landon MB, Spong CY, Thom E, et al.; National Institute of Child Health and Human Development Maternal-Fetal Medicine Units Network. Risk of uterine rupture with a trial of labor in women with multiple and single prior cesarean delivery. Obstet Gynecol. 2006;108:12-20.

6. Macones GA, Cahill A, Pare E, et al. Obstetric outcomes in women with two prior cesarean deliveries: is vaginal birth after cesarean delivery a viable option? Am J Obstet Gynecol. 2005;192:1223-8; discussion 1228-9.

7. Miller DA, Diaz FG, Paul RH. Vaginal birth after cesarean: a 10-year experience. Obstet Gynecol. 1994;84:255-8.

8. Spaans WA, van der Vliet LM, Röell-Schorer EA, et al. Trial of labour after two or three previous caesarean sections. Eur J Obstet Gynecol Reprod Biol. 2003;110:16-9.

9. Royal College of Obstetricians and Gynaecologists. Birth After Previous Caesarean Birth. Green-top Guideline No. 45 October 2015. London: RCOG.

10. Chimpf MO, Rahn DD, Wheeler TL, et al. Sling surgery for stress urinary incontinence in women: a systematic review and metaanalysis. Am J Obstet Gynecol. 2014;211(1):71.e171.e27.

11. Rovner ES, Wein AJ. Drug treatment of voiding dysfunction. In: Cardozo L, Staskin D (Eds). Textbook of Female Urology and Urogynecology, 1st edition. London: Isis Medical Media; 2001. pp. 357-407.

12. Martlew VJ. Peri-operative management of patients with coagulation disorders. Br J Anaesth. 2000;85(3):446-55.

5

Communication with Patients

'Medicine is an art whose magic and creative ability have long been recognized as residing in the interpersonal aspects of patient-physician relationship.'[1]

INTRODUCTION

Effective communication between the doctor and the patient is of prime importance for building a therapeutic relationship between doctor and the patient.[1] A satisfying patient-doctor relationship guarantees delivery of high-quality healthcare.[2]

Much of the patients' dissatisfaction and many grievances occur due to the failure of the doctor-patient relationship. A doctor who possesses the appropriate communication and interpersonal skills is likely to collect sufficient information from the patients. This information not only helps the clinicians in establishing an accurate diagnosis, but also offering appropriate counselling and therapeutic instructions, and establishing an empathetic relationship with patients.[3-5]

COMMUNICATION STATIONS

Communication skills for a doctor are extremely important in clinical practice while interacting with the patients. Though, there may be many stations in the MRCOG examination which would be testing the candidate's communication skills along with other core skills, some stations may focus exclusively on the candidate's communication skills. At ST5 level, the candidate would be communicating not only with the patients and their caretakers, but also with the colleagues, both junior and senior. Communication with the colleagues occurs at a level distinct from that occurring between the doctor and their patients. Therefore, it is discussed separately in details in Chapter 6.

Communication with the colleagues and communication with the patients can be different in several ways. While counselling the patient, it is important to make minimal use of medical terminology. The patient must be explained about the situation in as simple way as possible. Use of medical jargon must be at the minimum. The doctor should ascertain that the patients are able to comprehend the details related to their management which are explained to them. The candidate can draw simple diagrams to help the role-player understand a particular situation. During every patient-doctor interaction, the candidate is expected to demonstrate the following skills enumerated in Box 5.1.

While some OSCE stations during the MRCOG part 3 examination would be purely counselling stations, others may have 'counselling' as one of the component.

COUNSELLING SKILLS

At these stations, the examiner is mainly marking the candidates for the way they interact with the role-player and their counselling skills. Clinical knowledge in such stations is often secondary. The role-player may have been trained to display different kind of emotions. They may act as if they are sad or angry or upset. A competent candidate will be able to bring the situation under control by successfully counselling and reassuring the patient. If the 'patient' is angry, the competent candidates would allow her to talk and vent out her feelings. At the same time, they would keep the situation in control by adequately consoling the patient. The candidate must not personally take the feelings exhibited by the role-player at any point. They have been trained

---

BOX 5.1: Key skills which must highlight any patient-doctor communication.

- Starting any meeting with a suitable introduction explaining their name, role, and purpose of interaction
- Establishing an appropriate rapport with the patient
- Taking a concise, relevant history using a combination of open and closed questions. However, the open questions must be primarily used along with a few closed questions. The doctor must follow a logical and a clearly reasoned style of questioning
- The doctor must follow an empathetic approach, actively listening, and responding to the patient cues
- Identification and management of communication barriers, including the use of interpreters
- Providing information in small volumes using patient-friendly language. Use of medical jargon must be avoided and clinical terms must be explained
- Promoting dialogue with the patient and encouraging shared decision-making
- Demonstrating respect for patient autonomy in decision-making including when decisions are made against medical advice
- Accepting and addressing patient's concerns
- Ability of taking informed consent from the patient and demonstrating the awareness of mental capacity
- Ensuring suitable use of chaperones, especially during intimate examination
- Maintaining patient dignity and privacy at all times and being sensitive to cultural and religious issues

to behave that way in order to test the candidate. If the role-player becomes upset or tearful and starts sobbing, the candidate must display an empathetic and compassionate attitude towards her. The candidate must let her talk and patiently listen to her. It is a good idea to offer her tissues if she becomes tearful during the conversation.

Breaking Bad News

An important part of communicating with the patient is breaking bad news. This could be involved in a wide variety of MRCOG part 3 scenarios such as diagnosis of anencephaly, Down syndrome or some other congenital malformation or an intrauterine death or a stillbirth in obstetrics stations. In gynaecological stations, breaking bad news may be in form of disclosing the diagnosis of malignancy or diagnosis of some post-operative complication or failed surgery.

The candidate attempting MRCOG part 3 is expected to display empathy while breaking bad news to the role-player. They must also show appropriate emotional responses based on the responses given by the role-player. The role-player may have been instructed to start sobbing while the candidate breaks bad news to them. Though in general at most of the MRCOG part 3 stations, the candidate is expected to give a small smile to the actor as well as the examiner, it is best to curb one's smile while delivering bad news. The candidate should preferably adopt an empathic, patient-centred approach in these scenarios. They need to deal the situation with care and compassion, at the same time not concealing the truth. Since the news can be typically devastating for the patient, it is important to refrain from saying words such as 'okay' and 'alright'. At the same time, the candidates must also carefully observe if the role-player actually understands what they are trying to say.

If the role-player becomes tearful on hearing the bad news, the candidate must pause briefly. They must offer her tissues and ask her if she is alright. A competent candidate would also ask the patient if some of her relative or friend is accompanying her and would she want them to be present with her. The candidates must remember that during the examination the actor has been instructed to become tearful just to test them. The actors just want to see their behaviour.

While practicing such stations with an exam buddy, it is best for the candidate to get themselves videoed in order to visualise themselves for evaluating their unconscious expression while delivering bad news. They can even practice with their senior colleagues who may be able to point-out their unconscious behaviour as well as provide them with a valuable feedback.

Taking Consent

Communication with patients in the practice of obstetrics and gynaecology requires a different level of skills because many of the patients (e.g. obstetric patients or those making contraceptive choices) do not fit into the 'sick patient' role.

Therefore, in these cases the doctors must develop the ability to inform, engage, negotiate, and make shared decisions with the patients.

Before carrying out any surgical procedure in the patient, it is the duty of the doctor to take informed consent. Today, the informed consent is required for all operative procedures. The process involves counselling the patient about the various available surgical options so that the patient can select the best surgical procedure out of the various available options. In practice, the informed consent involves informing the patient about the diagnosis, degree of certainty regarding the diagnosis, the surgery that would be recommended in that case and possible alternatives along with their expected outcomes, and risks and benefits. The patient outcome, if no therapy is administered, must also be explained to the patient. The consent should be taken well in advance of surgery in a comfortable setting. The patient must be given adequate time to absorb the information, ask any questions if she feels so and then to make an informed decision. Effective communication between the patient and the surgeon is of utmost importance, while counselling the patient regarding various available treatment options. The surgeon may make use of written material (self-explanatory patient leaflets), visual aids (models), websites, etc. to explain the procedure to the patients. The patients must also be informed about the advantages, disadvantages, success and failure rates, and complications of the various procedures. The patient must be counselled even regarding the rare complications that are serious and may affect the individual's life. The informed consent requires the presence of following pieces of information: nature of the procedure; rationale of doing the procedure; advantages and disadvantages of doing the procedure; and availability of alternatives. The elements of informed consent are as follows:

- Disclosure of information
- Comprehension by the patient
- Voluntary transaction
- Validation.

Disclosure of Information

The patients must be explained about their diagnosis and also briefed about the various available treatment options, including no treatment, and various medical, surgical and alternative therapies. Risks and benefits of each modality need to be explained in sufficient details so that a reasonable adult patient can understand the situation and make an informed choice.

Comprehension by the Patient

The language and the descriptive material, which is used to explain the situation to the patient, must be appropriate to the patient's level of comprehension. The patients must be asked questions in-between to ensure that they have understood what they have been told.

Voluntariness

While making a decision, the patient must be free of coercion or constraints and must be able to choose freely. The patient should be mentally competent to be able to make a choice and there must be no evidence of limitation in her ability to understand the information. She must be in a condition to act independently on the basis of information that has been disclosed.

Validation

A written consent form must be given to the patient, which must be duly signed by her. Consent must be taken for each procedure, which is going to be performed even if they are being performed in a single sitting. If an additional pathology is discovered at the time of surgery, the surgeon can legally operate on it, only if the condition is life-threatening. On the other hand, if the condition is not life-threatening, then the surgeon must finish the planned surgery and discuss the condition later with the patient.

OSCE STATION 1: CONGENITAL ANOMALY

Candidate's Instructions

You are the registrar in the Department of Obstetrics and Gynaecology. Mrs Kay Barker, aged 29 years and pregnant for the first time, has come for a routine anomaly scan at 20 weeks of gestation. During this scan, the foetus is found to have a diaphragmatic hernia. She has been informed of the abnormality by the radiographer. The radiographer has called you to confirm the diagnosis and offer counselling regarding the prenatal diagnosis. You agree with the radiographer's diagnosis. How will you go about managing this patient?

The task is for 12 minutes (inclusive of 2 minutes of reading time). You have 10 minutes to counsel her about the situation. You shall be awarded marks for the following tasks:

Candidate's tasks:

- Explaining the diagnosis to the patient
- Discussing the management options with the patient
- Discussing the investigations required in this case
- Dealing with the patient's concerns.

These tasks cover the domains as discussed next.

Core Clinical Skills Domains

Core clinical skills domains tested:

- Communication with patients
- Information gathering
- Application of knowledge.

Module Tested

The module tested in this station is Module 4 or 'Antenatal Care'.

Role-player's Brief

- You are Mrs Kay Barker, a 29-year-old woman who has been referred for a routine anomaly scan at 20 weeks. You are in good spirits because of your pregnancy and you feel that nothing can go wrong. You think that the scan is a just a routine one and merely a formality.
- However, in the middle of the scan you realise that something is not quite right, because the radiographer has called a doctor who has taken you to a separate consultation room to discuss things. You are obviously scared and surprised because you never expected this.
- The doctor will tell you that your baby is suffering from malformations in the diaphragm, which may or may not be compatible with life. Diaphragm is a muscle which separates chest from the abdomen. Medically, the defect, which your baby suffers from, is diaphragmatic hernia. If the doctor just tells you the medical terms, ask for further explanation of these defects. You will question the doctor about the various options available to you, including termination and continuation of pregnancy. You are naturally upset about the situation.
- You are a fervent Roman Catholic and need to see your priest and partner before you make any decision. You ask about the possibility of treatment of the defect in case you decide to carry the pregnancy till term.
- This is your first pregnancy and your entire antenatal period had been uneventful. You had been trying to become pregnant since a past few months. Otherwise you are fit and well and there is no family history of any significant diseases.

Prompt Questions

- What are the various therapeutic options available to me?
- Is there requirement of further tests and/or a second opinion to help decide whether I should continue with the pregnancy or not.
- What is the possibility of treatment of the defect in case I decide to carry the pregnancy till term?
- Will my future pregnancies be affected with this defect?

EXAMINER'S INSTRUCTIONS AND STRUCTURED MARK SHEET

The examiner will mark the candidate on the basis of various tasks which are allotted to the candidate. Out of a total score of 20, the examiner can award a maximum of 18 marks, which are distributed between various candidate tasks as shown next. The role-player can award a maximum of 2 marks to the candidate. Each candidate task must be globally scored by the examiner.

Explaining the Diagnosis

- Does the candidate use a simple language, avoiding medical jargon to explain the defects? Diaphragmatic hernia is a hole in the flat muscles, separating the chest from the abdomen. You can draw simple diagrams to explain the defect to the patient (Fig. 5.1).

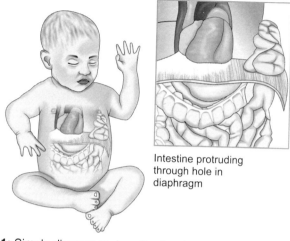

Intestine protruding
through hole in
diaphragm

Fig. 5.1: Simple diagram to describe the defect present in congenital diaphragmatic hernia.

- Does the candidate ask her if she wants her partner or relative to be called to come and join her? In case the role-player says that she wants time to discuss things with her partner and would come back at a later date with her decision, she should be given that option.
- Does the candidate explain the diagnosis to the patient and its possible implications? Congenital diaphragmatic hernia (CDH) may be a life-threatening situation in some cases. However, in some cases surgery can be performed following the baby's birth and the defect can be repaired.
- Does the candidate put the patient at ease and deal with her using care and compassion, thereby allowing her to express her concerns, shock, and confusion?
- Does the candidate explain the need for exclusion of other associated subtle structural and chromosomal abnormalities?

Marking Scheme

0	1	2	3	4
Fail		Borderline		Pass

Discussing the Management Options

- Offers option of either termination or continuing pregnancy.
- She can be offered paediatric consultation to help her take the decision if she so desires.

Termination

- According to the Abortion Act 1967 (amended Human Fertilisation and Embryology Act 1990), if the congenital abnormality is incompatible

with extrauterine life, abortions done under this criteria are legal beyond 24 weeks of gestation.[6]
- *Mode of termination*: Intracardiac potassium chloride can be injected depending on the period of gestation.
- Various methods for abortion are enumerated in Figure 5.2. Medical abortion can be performed using a combination of oral mifepristone tablets and gemeprost vaginal pessaries in the dosage based on the local protocols. If this method is not successful, medication can be introduced in the extra-amniotic space using an extra-amniotic Foley's catheter. However, in these cases, there may be a requirement for uterine evacuation following the procedure.
- In cases of induced medical abortion, the woman may experience pain similar to that of labour pains. Therefore, pain relief may be required in these cases.
- The patient needs to sign the consent form before getting on with the process.
- Offer post-mortem examination of the aborted baby.
- Offer photos, hand and foot prints of the aborted baby.

Continuation of Pregnancy
- Routine antenatal care would need to be undertaken
- Prenatal foetal karyotype analysis is required in order to rule out any chromosomal anomaly in the foetus.
- In some cases, it is possible to repair the defect on the diaphragm (Figs. 5.3A to C). It is important to decide the place of delivery in these cases. Delivery would be required in a perinatal centre with level 3 paediatric

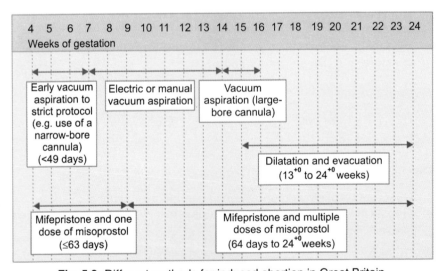

Fig. 5.2: Different methods for induced abortion in Great Britain.

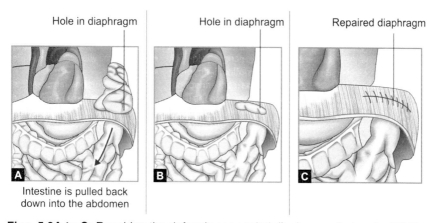

Figs. 5.3A to C: Repairing the defect in congenital diaphragmatic hernia: (A) The intestines are pulled down through the defect in the diaphragm; (B) The defect in the diaphragm is repaired; (C) Appearance of diaphragm following the repair of the defect.

ICU having neonatal and paediatric support. There should be availability of obstetricians/perinatologists, neonatologists, and paediatric surgeons so that the baby can be stabilised as well as treated.[7] There should be facilities for extracorporeal membrane oxygenation.

Marking Scheme

0	1	2	3	4	5
Fail		Borderline		Pass	

Investigations

In cases of CDH, it is important to determine the type of defect, its severity, and other associated defects to detect if the abnormality is a part of a syndrome. If the abnormality is a part of a syndrome, it is likely to be more severe. CDH may be associated with other major structural anomalies and chromosomal abnormalities. The chromosomal abnormalities most commonly associated with CDH include trisomy 21, 18, and 13.[8] Other complex structural chromosomal abnormalities are translocations, deletions, duplications, and marker chromosomes. CDH has also been reported in association with multiple syndromes such as Pallister-Killian syndrome, Fryns syndrome, DiGeorge syndrome, Apert syndrome, etc.[9,10] Structural anomalies such as congenital heart defects, neural tube defects (hydrocephalus, anencephaly, and spina bifida), hydronephrosis, renal agenesis, intestinal atresia, etc. may be associated with CDH.[8] Various investigations which may be required in these cases include level II ultrasound, echocardiogram, MRI, etc. Therefore, further scanning at tertiary level, foetomaternal medicine unit, is required in these cases.

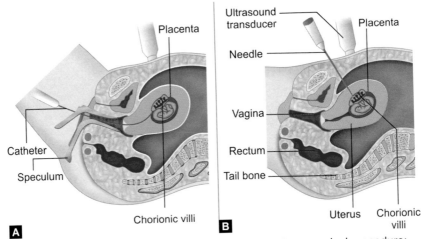

Figs. 5.4A and B: Chorionic villus sampling: (A) Transcervical procedure; (B) Transabdominal procedure.

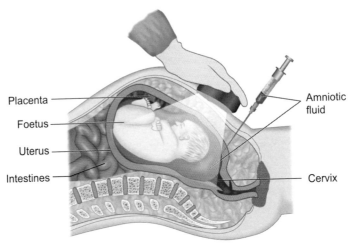

Fig. 5.5: Diagrammatic representation of the procedure of amniocentesis.

Prenatal karyotyping: Prenatal karyotype analysis is required for the detection on any underlying chromosomal abnormality and for the assessment of the disease severity. Chorionic villus sampling (CVS) (Figs. 5.4A and B) is performed most commonly between 11 weeks to 13 weeks of gestation. Amniocentesis (Fig. 5.5) is performed after 15 weeks, usually between 16 weeks to 20 weeks of gestation. The advantages and disadvantages of both the procedures need to be explained. The additional overall risk of miscarriage from amniocentesis is approximately 1% and that with CVS is about 1–2%.[11] Both amniocentesis and CVS can be done in combination with fluorescent in situ hybridisation (FISH).

The major advantage of this combination is that FISH serves as a swift method for counting the number of certain chromosomes within cells. Due to this, it can give faster results if used on an amniocentesis sample. While standard amniocentesis may give results within 2–3 weeks, FISH provides results within 24–48 hours. A normal FISH test has an accuracy of about 98% in predicting that a baby is likely to have a normal chromosome result. The major disadvantage with FISH is that it involves the use of only specific probes, and therefore other uncommon karyotypic abnormalities may not be excluded.

Marking Scheme

0	1	2	3	4	5
Fail		Borderline		Pass	

Understanding the Patient Concerns

- The patient must be asked if she needs time to think before she takes a decision. She should be given the option of thinking over and coming back after some time with the decision.
- In case she chooses termination of pregnancy, post-mortem examination may be a useful option.
- Arrange for any appropriate counselling both before and after delivery.
- Appropriate bereavement counselling must be provided to the patient.
- *Consequences for a future pregnancy*: Rate of recurrence of CDH depends on whether it occurs as an isolated finding, as part of a genetic syndrome or chromosome abnormality, or as part of a complex but non-syndromic set of findings. In case of genetic syndrome, rate of recurrence of CDH depends on the pattern of inheritance (autosomal dominant, autosomal recessive or sex-linked recessive). In isolated cases, the risk of recurrence is usually low between 1% to 2%.

Marking Scheme

0	1	2	3	4
Fail		Borderline		Pass

Role-player's Score

The role-player can award a maximum of 2 marks to the candidate.

Marking Scheme

0	1	2
Role-player never wants to see candidate again	Role-player prepared to see candidate again	Role-player happy to see candidate again

Total score: /20

DISCUSSION

Issues

At this station, the candidate is expected to break the bad news concerning the presence of life-threatening congenital malformation in the baby and to offer counselling regarding prenatal diagnosis. Marks would be awarded for candidate's ability to communicate with the role-player in a simple language, avoiding the use of medical jargon. The role-player has already been explained the scenario. She may become angry or upset depending on the situation. She, however, will not swear or shout at the candidate. If the candidate is going on a wrong tract, the role-player may give an indirect cue so that the candidate comes back on the track. Therefore, it is important for the candidate to closely follow what the role-player is trying to say. She has been given key points to test candidates' ability to apply their knowledge in a particular clinical situation. The role-player will give score to the patient, which can vary from 0 to 2. This score reflects how a patient would have evaluated the candidate in a normal clinical scenario if she had been treated by him/her.

Pitfalls

The major difficulty faced by the candidates in all counselling questions is that they fail to read the question properly and as a result do not answer it correctly. The 'candidate's instructions' described at the entry of each OSCE station must be carefully read by the candidate. If the instructions suggest that the diagnosis is clear and the candidate is just supposed to break the bad news to the role-player, as is the case in the above-mentioned OSCE station, then they must just do that. In that case, the candidates must not waste their time in taking the patient's history. In most of the scenarios associated with breaking bad news, there will be no doubt about the diagnosis. In these scenarios, the candidate shall be awarded marks for dealing with the situation and not for taking history, establishing diagnosis or formulating a management plan.

In this case, the patient is a Roman Catholic and may want to consult her priest and husband before taking a decision. If she asks for some time so that she can discuss things with her husband and priest and come back at a later date, she should be allowed to do so. Asking the patient to take a decision instantly can also be considered as a potential error.

Variations

In the obstetric scenario, there can be variable scenarios varying from breaking bad news about a rare congenital anomaly (fatal or non-fatal) to that of breaking bad news regarding a more common one (e.g. Down syndrome). Another common scenario on obstetric stations may be breaking bad news regarding an IUD or still birth. When you are preparing for the MRCOG Part 3 examination, make sure you also practice regarding these scenarios with your exam buddy because these can be commonly asked in the examination.

OSCE STATION 2: BREAKING BAD NEWS RELATED TO THE PRESENCE OF MALIGNANCY

Candidate's Instructions

You are the registrar in the gynaecological outpatient clinic and you are about to see Ms Joan Dunn, a 30-year-old single woman, who is a teacher by profession. She has been largely asymptomatic. She was referred for colposcopy on account of a severe dyskaryotic smear obtained at the time of routine cervical sample screening. At the time of colposcopy, colposcopic-directed biopsy was also taken. The results of the biopsy have come and she has been called to obtain the results. You have to give her the report and explain her, the diagnosis. Shown below is her histopathology report. Please counsel Ms Dunn.

Leighton Hospital,
Crewe, Cheshire
Department of Pathology

Histopathology report

Patient name: Joan Dunn
ID no.: P7861264
Age: 30 year
Date: 28 December 2016
Specimen: Small amount of cervical tissue (removed under colposcopic guidance)
Histology report: Moderately differentiated squamous cell carcinoma of the cervix

Validated by: Dr Ruby Merchant (MRC Path)

The task is for 12 minutes (inclusive of 2 minutes of reading time). You have 10 minutes to counsel her about the situation. Marks would be awarded for the following tasks:

Candidate's tasks:
- Taking the relevant patient's history
- Breaking the bad news and explaining her the diagnosis
- Discussing the management options with the patient and dealing with her concerns.

These tasks cover the domains as discussed next.

Core Clinical Skills Domains

Core clinical skills domains tested:
- Communication with patients
- Information gathering
- Application of knowledge.

Module Tested

The module tested in this station is Module 13 or 'Gynaecological Oncology'.

Role-player's Brief

- You are Ms Joan Dunn, a 30-year-old woman, who is a primary school teacher by profession. You are presently single but you are engaged with

John, a business executive by profession. You are likely to be married within the coming 6 months. You love kids and would love to have at least two kids with John. Presently, you stay with your parents. Your family is financially stable. You have good family support and share a decent relationship with your parents and siblings.

- You feel you would be reasonably rich after marriage. You are very happy with life and want to spend rest of your life taking care of your husband and children.
- Your first period (menarche) was at the age of 10 year. Your periods have largely been regular with each cycle lasting for 20–30 days. Your periods last for 4–5 days and are not heavy. You have mild, tolerable dysmenorrhoea. You have always thought this pattern of periods was normal.
- You have never experienced any intermenstrual bleeding or bleeding in between periods. You also have not experienced bleeding after sexual activity.
- You have not taken any regular medication including oral contraceptive agents in the past.
- As a teenager you have had a few one-night stands in the past but you always remembered to use a condom. Your first stable relationship was with John and you have been in a stable sexual relationship with him since past 3 years. Now, John is the only one for you and you think John also feels the same.
- You smoke about 20 cigarettes per day, and drink alcohol socially on occasions.
- You and your partner have not suffered from any sexually transmitted diseases in the past.
- There is no medical or surgical history.
- There is no family history of any cancers.
- There is no history of any allergies.
- Fifteen days back you had a routine cervical smear done. You felt this was a routine as you have been getting the cervical smears done since the age of 25 years. You became slightly worried because the doctor found an abnormality on the smear and referred you for colposcopy. A biopsy was taken at the time of colposcopy and you have been called to receive the biopsy result. Now you are really scared because you are anticipating the worst. You are worried about the result of the biopsy.
- Initially when the doctor tells you about the news of having a cancer, you are not ready to believe it. You feel you have been told about the wrong results. You believe that a cancer is very painful and you have never had any symptoms.
- When the doctor tries to convince you about the diagnosis of cancer, you get extremely upset after knowing about the cancer, especially when you are to be married and plan to have children.

Prompt Questions

- What is the result of the biopsy, doctor?
- How can it be cancer? I never had any symptoms.

- Is the cancer curable? Why has this happened to me?
- How successful is the surgery in curing the disease doctor?
- Is there no way for me to have children in the future?
- What are the risks of the surgery?

EXAMINER'S INSTRUCTIONS AND STRUCTURED MARK SHEET

The examiner will mark the candidate on the basis of various tasks which are allotted to the candidate. Out of a total score of 20, the examiner can award a maximum of 18 marks, which are distributed between various candidate tasks as shown next. The role-player can award a maximum of 2 marks to the candidate. Each candidate task must be globally scored by the examiner.

Relevant Patient's History

- *Menstrual history*: Previous history of regular menstrual cycles. No history of any intermenstrual or post-coital bleeding.
- *Risk factors*: No obvious history of promiscuous behaviour with the patient or her partner; had a few one-night stands as a teenager; used condom; in a stable relationship since past 3 years. There is no history of sexually transmitted diseases.
- *Family history*: There is no family history of any cancers.
- *Future fertility requirements*: To be married in 6 months and plans to have children.
- *Social support*: Belongs to a financially stable family and has good family support.
- No past medical or surgical history.
- Smokes about 20 cigarettes in a day.
- Drinks alcohol socially on occasions.

Marking Scheme

0	1	2	3	4	5
Fail		Borderline		Pass	

Breaking the Bad News and Explaining the Diagnosis

- Offers counselling to cope up with news.
- Follows the previously mentioned precautions while breaking bad news.
- She might be shocked after being told about the diagnosis of malignancy in the neck of the womb (cervix). Deal her with compassion and empathy.
- She should be given the option of calling her friend or relatives, if she so desires before breaking the bad news to her.
- She should be reassured that quality assurance procedures are in place in the histopathology laboratory to ensure that the correct diagnosis is made.
- Extent of disease is presently unknown; she would require staging, which is clinical in cases of cervical cancer.

- She will need further evaluation and tests (e.g. MRI and other imaging tests).
- Discussion of both imaging and pathology results would be required at a multidisciplinary team meeting to decide further course of management.

Marking Scheme

0	1	2	3	4	5
Fail		Borderline		Pass	

Discussing the Management Options

- She must be advised to stopping smoking because smoking is likely to affect the local immunity in the cervix and acts as a risk factor for cancer development.
- She can consult her general practitioner (GP) or the National Health Service (NHS) Stop Smoking Services to help her quit smoking.
- Prognosis depends on the results of cancer staging. For stage IA (microinvasive cervical cancer), the 5-years survival rate is about 93%; for stage IB (early stage cervical cancer), the 5-year survival rate is about 80%.[12]
- Clinical staging will help to determine her treatment options.
- Clinical staging would involve examination under anaesthesia (parametrial, vaginal and rectal examination, and cystoscopy) and radiological investigations to exclude distant metastases (chest X-ray; magnetic resonance imaging; ultrasound scans of the abdomen and urinary tract).
- If the woman with a microinvasive disease desires future fertility, the options to be considered include cone biopsy and trachelectomy.
- Conisation with clear margins may be considered adequate in young patients with stage IA disease who want to conserve their uterus. For effective treatment, there must not be any evidence of lymphovascular space invasion and both endocervical margins and curettage findings must be negative for cancer or dysplasia.
- The patients undergoing conisation require close follow-up, including cytology, colposcopy, and endocervical curettage.
- In young women desirous of childbearing, conservative treatment comprising of laparoscopic lymphadenectomy followed by vaginal trachelectomy can be done.
- Radical trachelectomy is rapidly emerging as a surgical management option in women with stage IA2 and IB1 disease who desire preservation of uterus and fertility.[13,14]
- It is important to counsel the patient that these treatment strategies are still under the research stages. Although preliminary results in some centres are encouraging, long-term follow-up in a large series is not yet available.
- Women who are able to conceive after surgery are likely to develop preterm labour or late miscarriages.
- For early invasive disease (stage Ia2–IIa), a Wertheim's hysterectomy followed by adjuvant radiotherapy, if the nodes are involved, is the treatment of choice.[15]

- Wertheim's hysterectomy involves an abdominal hysterectomy, removal of the parametrium, pelvic nodes, and vaginal cuff (usually the upper third of the vagina).
- The major advantage of this surgery is that is allows preservation of the ovaries. So there is an option to conceive using the uterus of a surrogate mother.
- Complications of premature menopause are thus avoided. In addition, gynatresia, which is a complication of radiation, is absent.
- Surgical procedure, if required would be performed under general anaesthesia, midline incision would be required. She also needs to be counselled regarding the risks of surgery, i.e. anaesthetic risks, venous thromboembolism, bladder, bowel injury, bleeding, infection, etc.
- Subsequent management after will depend on the presence of positive nodes.
- If the nodes are negative, no additional (adjuvant) therapy is required.
- However, if the nodes are involved, radiotherapy, usually in the form of external beam radiation, is the adjunctive treatment of choice.
- For advanced disease (stages IIb–IIIa), radiotherapy, both external and intracavitary, can be administered.
- Once diagnosis of cancer has been made, then there is a 31-day target to commence treatment (Fig. 5.6).[16]

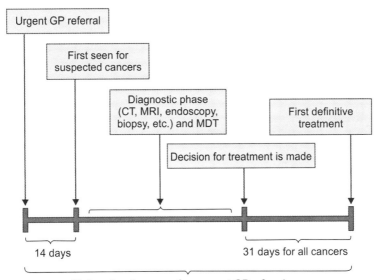

Fig. 5.6: Standard cancer waiting times. (GP: general practitioner; MDT: multi-disciplinary team; CT: computed tomography; MRI: magnetic resonance imaging)

Source: Department of health. (2008). Ensuring Better Treatment: Going Further on Cancer Waits. An improvement guide for supporting sustainable delivery. [online] Available from https://www.england.nhs.uk/wp-content/uploads/2015/03/going-further-cancer-waits.pdf [Accessed November 2017].

Marking Scheme

0	1	2	3	4	5
Fail		Borderline		Pass	

Dealing with her Concerns

- Helping her cope up with the situation.
- Addressing her concerns regarding future fertility.
- Her future fertility may not be affected with conservative management. However there may be increased chances of premature labour or late miscarriages.

Marking Scheme

0	1	2	3
Fail	Borderline		Pass

Role-player's Score

The role-player can award a maximum of 2 marks to the candidate.

Marking Scheme

0	1	2
Role-player never wants to see candidate again	Role-player prepared to see candidate again	Role-player happy to see candidate again

Total score: /20

DISCUSSION

Issues

This station tests the candidate's ability to break bad news to an unsuspecting patient, who had a cervical smear examination as part of the routine screening programme. She was referred for colposcopy and directed biopsy due to suspected suspicious smear. She had been completely asymptomatic. Disclosure of the diagnosis of cervical cancer can be particularly traumatic in this case. The candidate has to be particularly emphatic to such a patient while breaking bad news about diagnosis of a malignancy. The candidate should patiently address all her concerns, especially those related to the next course of management and future fertility. The patient in this case is young and is likely to be married in the coming months so she is likely to be particularly concerned about her ability to conceive. The stage of her cancer can only be confirmed after a clinical staging process and results of imaging. In cases of microinvasive or early stage cancer, conservative treatment is possible.

Pitfalls

The candidate must carefully read the tasks they are required to do. They have to take the patient's history as well as break the bad news. The station also requires them to explain the diagnosis, discuss the management options, and address the patient's concerns. It is particularly important for the candidate to divide their time so that they are able to cover all the aspects. Missing to cover a particular aspect of this station may prove to be disastrous.

The candidate must focus on the conservative management and also briefly describe about other modalities of treatment because the cancer stage is yet not clear in the given scenario. The fact that the conservative management is still under research stages needs to be emphasised.

Variations

This station is concerned with breaking bad news about the diagnosis of cervical cancer to an unsuspecting patient. There could be similar stations with different other types of cancers (e.g. endometrial cancer, ovarian cancer, vulvar cancer, etc.). The patients' concerns may vary in each scenario. Some may wish to conserve their fertility, or uterus or some just their ovaries. There might be no patient concerns and the station may be just focussing on testing your counselling skills and ability to break bad news.

OSCE STATION 3: COMMUNICATION SKILLS—FAILED PROCEDURE (ECTOPIC PREGNANCY REMAINS INTACT)

Candidate's Instructions

You are the registrar on duty and have been called to see a patient, Mrs Veronica Morgan, a 35-year-old woman, who has been referred to the hospital's early pregnancy unit (EPU) for follow-up by GP in lieu of continuing abdominal pain and vaginal bleeding. A salpingostomy for an ectopic pregnancy was performed in this patient 2 weeks ago. Following discharge, she continued to experience abdominal pain and vaginal bleeding especially on the left side. She had been called for a follow-up visit, 1 week following salpingostomy. However, she failed to come for that visit. Today, an ultrasound examination and blood levels of β-human chorionic gonadotropin (hCG) were performed. The ultrasound done today has shown a live ectopic pregnancy on the left side. You have been called to counsel Mrs Morgan and explain the ultrasound findings and the likely diagnosis. The task is for 12 minutes (inclusive of 2 minutes of reading time). You have 10 minutes to counsel her about the situation. Marks would be awarded to the candidate for the following tasks:

Candidate's tasks:

- Take relevant history and explain her the diagnosis
- Counsel the patient regarding the situation and address her concerns
- Suggest an appropriate management plan.

These tasks cover the domains as discussed next.

Core Clinical Skills Domains

Core clinical skills domains tested:

- Communication with patients
- Information gathering
- Application of knowledge
- Patient safety.

Module Tested

The module tested in this station is Module 12 or 'Early Pregnancy Care'.

Role-player's Brief

- You are Veronica Morgan, a 35-year-old woman, who is also a Jehovah's Witness (JW). You are a solicitor by profession. You are quite a bossy woman and you are used to being in charge and telling everyone what to do. You had your last menstrual period (LMP) 9 weeks ago. This is your second pregnancy. You and your partner had been particularly excited about this pregnancy.
- Your first pregnancy had turned out to be an ectopic pregnancy for which your right-sided tube was removed.
- You have no significant past medical or surgical history except that you had your appendix removed when you were about 12 years old.
- You had been trying to get pregnant since past 18 months. Your pregnancy has not been problematic since the beginning. You experienced some vaginal bleeding at about 6-7 weeks of gestation. At 7 weeks you presented to the EPU with severe abdominal pain. An ultrasound scan was performed and you were told that you had an ectopic pregnancy.
- You underwent a laparoscopy, where the tube was opened up and the ectopic pregnancy was removed. You were discharged home after 2 days and advised to return for a follow-up visit after a week. You were told that the levels of the pregnancy hormone (β-hCG) would be tested during this visit. However, ever since you have been discharged home, you have continued to experience abdominal pain and vaginal bleeding. You had generally not been feeling very well so you did not go to the hospital for the follow-up visit. Now, the pain has been getting severe on the left side. So you met your GP, who acted very quickly and you were readmitted to the hospital. The doctor performed another scan and did another blood test. You were made to wait nearly for an hour before you could have the scan and the blood test. You are quite irritated with the whole scenario and want to know what went wrong?
- You have not been yet told about the results of the scan or the blood test. However, you have been told that you would be meeting a doctor who would explain the scan results and further management.
- You will be told that the ectopic pregnancy is still present in your left tube. You are very angry about the situation because you had previously been

told that the tubal pregnancy had been removed. On the whole, you feel that your care was negligent. You want an explanation for your condition.

- You want to immediately meet the doctor who performed the surgery on you so that you can express your displeasure.
- You do not want your tube to be removed at any cost because you would want to conceive in the future. You want conservative treatment. Therefore, you are looking at a further laparoscopy.
- You are otherwise fit and well and you take no medications and do not smoke or drink alcohol. You have no family history of any significant diseases and you are not allergic to anything.
- You are a JW and are obstinate about not receiving any blood products.

Prompt Questions

- Why was my ectopic pregnancy not removed the first time when the surgery was performed 2 weeks ago?
- Was the person who performed the laparoscopy competent enough to be doing this on her own?
- I want to become pregnant in future. What are my available treatment options?
- I want to meet the doctor who performed the surgery on me.
- I plan to take this further. I want to register a complaint and seek legal ·advice. Whom do I contact?

EXAMINER'S INSTRUCTIONS AND STRUCTURED MARK SHEET

The examiner will mark the candidate on the basis of various tasks, which are allotted to the candidate. Out of a total score of 20, the examiner can award a maximum of 18 marks, which are distributed between various candidate tasks as shown next. The role-player can award a maximum of 2 marks to the candidate. The examiner must globally score each candidate task.

Taking the Relevant History and Explaining her the Diagnosis

- Checking her LMP.
- Checking her obstetric history till date; this is her second pregnancy; she conceived after 18 months of trying.
- Her first pregnancy turned out to be an ectopic pregnancy due to which salpingectomy on the right side was done.
- Current pregnancy was diagnosed as an ectopic and a laparoscopic salpingostomy was performed 2 weeks ago.
- She was advised to come for a follow-up visit after 1 week for monitoring the β-hCG levels, which she failed to attend.
- Ask her about the current symptoms.
- Explain that her ultrasound and blood reports have revealed an ectopic pregnancy.
- Ask her expectations about future pregnancy.

Marking Scheme

0	1	2	3	4	5	6
Fail		Borderline		Pass		

Counselling the Patient and Addressing her Concerns

- The patient is clearly upset about the situation, deal with her empathically.
- Apologise that the surgeon who had performed the laparoscopy is not available. Do not blame previous surgeon for supposed negligence.
- Explain that the specialist registrars (SpRs) are all competent and they have all been assessed on their competencies before undertaking a procedure such as laparoscopic management of ectopic pregnancy.
- There is always a designated consultant in the labour ward on duty. If the SpR faces any technical difficulties at the time of surgery, the consultant is called for help.
- Try to diffuse the situation by emphasising that salpingostomy may sometimes be associated with an inherent failure rate, therefore requires monitoring with β-hCG levels following surgery.
- Clarify that persistent ectopics can sometimes occur with laparoscopic conservative surgery for tubal ectopics.

Addressing the Patient's Concerns

- *The patient wants to register a formal complaint and seek legal advice. She needs to know whom she should contact?*
- She should be told about the process of registering a complaint in a neutral manner. She should be advised to register her complaint first and then seek legal advice.
- She should be advised to seek help from PALS (Patient Advice and Liaison Service). PALS serve as a point of contact for patients, their families, and their carers. It offers confidential advice, support, and information about health-related matters and the NHS complaints procedure.[17] Details of the nearest PALS can be obtained from the GP, or by calling NHS at 111.
- The patient can also complain to the commissioner of that service—either NHS England or the area Clinical Commissioning Group (CCG). While the most primary care services, such as GP and dental services, are commissioned by the NHS England; secondary care services, such as hospital care, are commissioned by the CCGs.
- She should be advised that since the case triggered a risk management alert, a full investigation would have been begun in the hospital unit involved.

Marking Scheme

0	1	2	3	4	5	6
Fail		Borderline		Pass		

Suggesting an Appropriate Management Plan

- There is requirement for another surgery, most likely laparoscopy.
- Surgery either in the form of salpingectomy (removal of the tube) or salpingotomy (cut in the tube to remove the ectopic) would be required.
- Salpingectomy results in the complete removal of the tube. Salpingectomy of one tube may reduce the chances of future conception. Salpingotomy and salpingostomy both are tube-conserving procedures (Figs. 5.7A and B). However, these procedures must be followed by regular monitoring of β-hCG levels to ensure that there is no remnant trophoblastic tissue.[18] Linear incision of the tubal wall, followed by suturing the wall after removal of the conceptus, is known as salpingotomy. In this case, the tubal closure occurs by primary intention. On the other hand, in salpingostomy, the initial steps are similar to that followed in salpingotomy. The only difference is that healing occurs by secondary intention in this case.
- Patient's wishes for conservative surgery in this case must be accepted.
- She should be told that in case she gets salpingectomy (Figs. 5.8A and B) done, in vitro fertilisation (IVF) would be the only option available for her to attain future fertility.
- She should be explained that ectopic pregnancy is a potentially life-threatening condition.
- Suggest that there may be a requirement for blood transfusion in case of sizeable blood loss.

Dealing with the aspect of JW: The patient is a JW and adamantly denies any kind of blood transfusion.
- In these cases, the patient's autonomy needs to be respected. It would be considered an assault to give a blood transfusion to JW against their wishes.

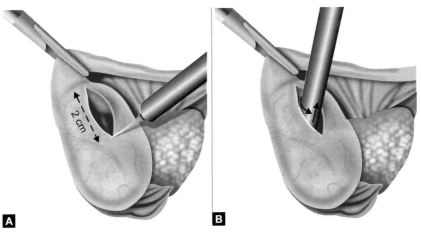

A **B**

Figs. 5.7A and B: Tube sparing salpingotomy: (A) A small incision given over the tubal ectopic; (B) Suction of the trophoblast tissue of the unruptured ectopic pregnancy.

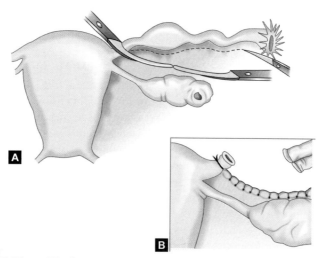

Figs. 5.8A and B: Salpingectomy: (A) Procedure of total salpingectomy at laparotomy; (B) Excision and suture ligation of the mesosalpinx at laparotomy.

If done so, the matter may be reported to the General Medical Council (GMC) or may be taken to the court.

- Respect and acknowledge the patient's decision of not receiving any blood transfusion.
- Emphasise the need to test for blood group and risk of isoimmunisation.
- Discuss that she would need to sign a separate consent form.
- The patient may seek help from a JW advocate.
- The possibility of autologous transfusion depending on her wishes must be discussed.
- Cell saver or intraoperative blood salvage should be used in theatre.[19]

Marking Scheme

0	1	2	3	4	5	6
Fail		Borderline		Pass		

Role-player's Score

The role-player can award a maximum of 2 marks to the candidate.

Marking Scheme

0	1	2
Role-player never wants to see candidate again	Role-player prepared to see candidate again	Role-player happy to see candidate again

Total score: /20

DISCUSSION

Issues

This is a difficult situation where your counselling and communication skills would be tested. This station presents with a situation where the woman is angry about the fact that surgery has not been correctly performed. This station tests the candidate's ability to console the patient and to diffuse a situation. At the same time the candidate should be careful not to badmouth their colleagues or the hospital. The candidate must avoid saying that the previous operation was not done correctly. Simultaneously, the candidate must not become defensive about the situation. With regard to the patient's anger, the best strategy would be to listen to her with compassion to help her get her grudges off her chest.

Once you are done with counselling the patient, you have to manage the case. She has once had conservative surgery in form of salpingostomy, 2 weeks back, which was not successful. Candidate must very clearly tell the patient that repeating the conservative surgery (salpingostomy or salpingotomy) is likely to be associated with a very small chance of persistent trophoblastic tissue. This may also be associated with a future risk of an ectopic. She must be explained that salpingectomy is likely to be best option for dealing with the persistent trophoblastic tissue. However, in case of salpingectomy, IVF would be the only option available to her to attain future pregnancy. Moreover, her wishes for conservative surgery must be regarded.

Pitfalls

Besides testing the candidate's communication and counselling skills, this station also tests the candidate's ability to elicit a proper history of the patient. Communication skills are particularly important because the candidate has to console a patient who is pretty angry about the situation. The candidate must not criticise the doctor or the hospital at any point of time.

There are several aspects in the history which need to be considered in this case: one, she desires future fertility; two, she has a previous history of right-sided salpingectomy; and three she is a JW. Failure to elicit either of the point at the time of taking history may cause the candidate to fail the examination. After considering all these aspects, elicited while taking history, the candidate needs to devise a management plan. She should be counselled regarding the prognosis for future pregnancies and how would it be possible to conceive in future.

The station also requires the candidate to address the patient's concerns. In this case the patient wants to seek legal help and file a complaint against the doctor and the hospital. She should be guided about the next step of action in a neutral manner.

Variations

Many variations are possible with this kind of station. There could be failure of any kind of surgery, e.g. pregnancy after sterilisation procedure, vault prolapse following an abdominal hysterectomy, failure to detect the complications, etc.

OSCE STATION 4: PREOPERATIVE COUNSELLING (COUNSELLING THE PATIENT ABOUT TO UNDERGO ABDOMINAL HYSTERECTOMY)

Candidate's Instructions

You are the registrar who would be responsible for today's operating list in your ward. Your consultant would be available in case of an emergency, but prefers not to be disturbed. While taking the preoperative ward round you come across a patient, Mrs Andrews Bryce, who is a 48-years-old woman with a history of multiple uterine fibroids. She is posted for abdominal hysterectomy today. You have examined her and found her body mass index as 25 kg/m². Per abdominal examination reveals a soft, slightly distended abdomen. Per vaginal examination shows the uterus to be soft, irregular, and 20 weeks in size. The task is for 12 minutes (inclusive of 2 minutes of reading time). You have 10 minutes to counsel her about the situation. You shall be awarded marks for the following tasks:

Candidate's tasks:
- Taking the relevant history
- Which appropriate investigations would you ensure have been done?
- Counselling her regarding surgery and the post-operative period.

These tasks cover the domains as discussed next.

Core Clinical Skills Domains

Core clinical skills domains tested:
- Communication with patients
- Information gathering
- Application of knowledge.

Module Tested

The modules tested in this station are Module 2 or 'Core Surgical Skills' and Module 3 or 'Post-operative Care'.

Role-player's Brief

- You are Mrs Andrews Bryce, a 48-year-old woman with a history of multiple uterine fibroids. You are posted for an abdominal hysterectomy (removal of the uterus) today.

- You have been having heavy periods lasting for approximately 10–15 days during each cycle since past 6 months. The periods are more or less regular. The bleeding sometimes occurs irregularly in between your periods when you are expected to be dry. You have to wear pads every day and are generally worried. Bleeding is also accompanied with severe abdominal pain. On the heavy days of your cycle, you soak nearly 5–6 pads per day.
- You had consulted your GP regarding this problem and he had advised you combined oral contraceptive pills and some painkillers. He also prescribed you some iron pills.
- Your bleeding was not controlled so you were referred to the hospital by your GP for an ultrasound examination. Ultrasound revealed a large fibroid on the top of uterus, $12 \times 8 \times 6$ cm in dimensions and several small fibroids varying between 1 cm to 2 cm in diameter in the inner lining of the uterus (submucosal).
- You had your last cervical smear done 3 years back and that was normal.
- You have not noticed any symptoms such as chest pain, shortness of breath, palpitations or weight loss in the past.
- You do not smoke and occasionally drink alcohol.
- You also underwent hysteroscopy and endometrial sampling, which did not show any endometrial abnormality.
- Your recent Hb level was 12.5 g/dL. Other blood parameters were within normal limits.
- You are generally friendly in nature and are keenly interested in knowing about the surgery. You usually remain calm, but may turn aggressive if you are treated with disrespect or are degraded. You are a busy professional woman and want to be treated with appropriate respect.
- You work as an assistant to a dentist and at times have an extremely hectic work schedule. Your heavy bleeding and abdominal pain interfere with your work schedule. You really want a permanent solution to your problems.
- After having a detailed discussion with your doctor and your husband, you had finally decided that the best option for you would be to undergo a total abdominal hysterectomy. During the discussion you had with your doctor, it was decided that your ovaries would be conserved unless there occurs some complication at the time of surgery which can only be rectified by its removal.
- Prior to last 6 months your periods had been extremely normal. You attained menarche at the age of 12 years. You usually had cycles lasting between 25 days to 30 days, with your periods lasting for 5–6 days. The blood flow was normal and you usually soaked 2–3 pads per day on the heavy days of your periods.
- You have one 16-year-old son, who stays away from you because he studies in the Boston University. You do not want to become pregnant in the future.
- There is no significant treatment history.
- You are allergic to Amoxil (amoxicillin), because the last time you were prescribed this drug, you developed a rash.

- There is no significant past medical or surgical history except that you were diagnosed with presenile dementia 2 years ago. However, now you feel that you do not suffer from any kind of memory loss.
- There is a family history of diabetes. Your father suffers from diabetes controlled with medication.
- Your surgery is planned for today.

Prompt Questions

- What would happen if my ovaries were also removed during the surgery?
- What should I expect would happen in the post-operative period?

EXAMINER'S INSTRUCTIONS AND STRUCTURED MARK SHEET

The examiner will mark the candidate on the basis of various tasks, which are allotted to the candidate. Out of a total score of 20, the examiner can award a maximum of 18 marks, which are distributed between various candidate tasks as shown next. The role-player can award a maximum of 2 marks to the candidate. Each candidate task must be globally scored by the examiner.

Taking the Relevant History

- What are her main symptoms?
- Details of intermenstrual bleeding
- Details of her heavy periods
- Any history of post-coital bleeding?
- Has she received any gonadotropin-releasing hormone (GnRH) analogues or iron tablets?
- Date of LMP
- Previous menstrual history
- History of previous cervical smears
- Previous obstetric history
- Family history
- Social history, including that of smoking, alcohol, and recreational drugs
- Past history of any medical illness, any allergies?
- Any previous surgery, especially abdominal?
- Have the various management options (surgical and conservative) been evaluated?
- Has the option of preserving the ovaries been discussed?
- Has the option of subtotal hysterectomy (Figs. 5.9A to C) been discussed?

Marking Scheme

0	1	2	3	4
Fail		Borderline		Pass

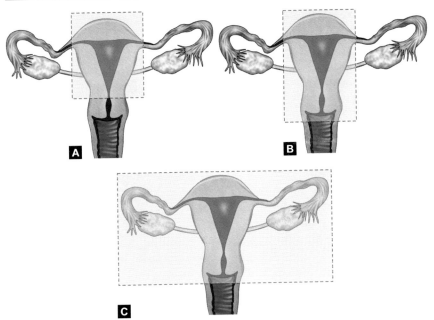

Figs. 5.9A to C: Different types of hysterectomy: (A) Subtotal hysterectomy where only the uterus and not the cervix is removed; (B) Total abdominal hysterectomy with conservation of ovaries; (C) Total abdominal hysterectomy with removal of both tubes and ovaries.

Ensuring the Relevant Investigations

- Ultrasound of the pelvis (including the uterus and the ovaries)
- Any available endometrial histology
- Full blood count
- Pregnancy test
- Cervical smear.

Marking Scheme

0	1	2	3	4
Fail		Borderline		Pass

Counselling her about Various Aspects of the Surgery

- Does she understand what kind of surgery she would be undergoing?
- Confirm if the ovarian conservation has been discussed?
- If ovaries are removed, the patient is likely to experience the symptoms of premature menopause. In these cases, hormone replacement therapy would be required.
- *Discuss the type of incision*: Vertical incision may be necessary because size of the uterus is increased in this case.

TABLE 5.1: Risks associated with hysterectomy.

Immediate	Intermediate	Long term
• Anaesthetic–risks due to general anaesthesia • Bladder or bowel injury • Haemorrhage	• DVT/PE • Bladder problems (e.g. voiding difficulties) • Infection	• DVT/PE • Bladder problems • Psychosexual, including loss of womanhood if ovaries are removed

(DVT: deep vein thrombosis; PE: pulmonary embolism)

- Would she opt for a subtotal hysterectomy or the total abdominal one?
- Subtotal hysterectomy is relatively easier to perform. It is associated with fewer post-operative complications such as bladder problems (e.g. voiding difficulty) and sexual function. However, since the cervix is retained in these cases, the patient may be at the risk of developing cervical carcinoma in future.
- Risks of likely complications related to total abdominal hysterectomy need to be explained to the patient; there may be a requirement for thromboprophylaxis post-operatively. Various complications associated with hysterectomy are tabulated in Table 5.1.
- Since there is a history of presenile dementia in this case, patient's capacity to give consent needs to be assessed by the doctor taking consent. The Mental Capacity Act, 2005, governs this. The candidate must ensure that the patient is able to comprehend and recall the information provided to her.

Marking Scheme

0	1	2	3	4	5
Fail		Borderline		Pass	

Post-operative Advice

- As the patient comes out of the operation theatre after the surgery, she is likely to have a tube attached to her arm (intravenous catheter). There is likely to be another tube to drain the urine from the urinary bladder (urinary catheter). Insertion of an intravenous line would ensure that adequate amount of intravenous fluids reach the patient. A urinary catheter, on the other hand, would enable the monitoring of the urine output at hourly intervals.
- Haemoglobin level would be checked to ensure she has not developed anaemia due to excessive blood loss during the surgery.
- There may be a possible requirement for an abdominal drain depending on the quantity of intraoperative blood loss.
- Requirement for thromboprophylaxis in the post-operative period.
- Precautions such as early mobilisation, foot and leg exercises and/or thromboembolic deterrent stockings.

Marking Scheme

0	1	2	3	4	5
Fail		Borderline		Pass	

Role-player's Score

The role-player can award a maximum of 2 marks to the candidate.

Marking Scheme

0	1	2
Role-player never wants to see candidate again	Role-player prepared to see candidate again	Role-player happy to see candidate again

Total score: /20

DISCUSSION

Issues

The candidate is required to carry out preoperative counselling in the patient who is about to undergo abdominal hysterectomy. Some issues, which must be particularly dealt with in such kind of station, are discussed next:

- Since a patient who has been experiencing heavy menstrual bleeding since past 3 months is likely to be anaemic, the candidate must remember to ask for the symptoms of anaemia while taking history. If the patient appears to be suffering from anaemia, the candidate should ensure that treatment for anaemia has been instituted preoperatively and she has a normal blood count prior to surgery. Although oral iron may prove to be sufficient, the discussion should also include prescription of hormonal ovarian suppressors (e.g. GnRH analogues), if oral iron therapy fails).
- Another important issue with this station is that the patient had been diagnosed to be suffering from presenile dementia. Thus her capacity to give consent needs to be assessed. This is governed by the Mental Capacity Act 2005.[20] The capacity of the patient to give a valid consent can be assessed in the four following ways:
  1. She is able to understanding the information provided to her
  2. She has the ability to retain that information
  3. She demonstrates the ability to decide on a particular issue
  4. She is able to communicate her understanding of the procedure.

  Sometimes, treatment can proceed without consent if it is in the patient's best interests. In this case, the patient's relatives or unpaid carers can be involved if the patient does not appear to understand the significance of the procedure.

Pitfalls

Inability to elicit the two above-described issues at the time of taking history can be considered as a possible fault.

This is a counselling station where the candidate's communication skills while counselling a patient regarding the operative and post-operative period would be assessed. The candidate should explain all the surgery-related details in a simplified manner. Use of medical jargon by the candidate is a potential pitfall and must be avoided at all costs. A good idea would be to go through the patient information leaflets describing various surgeries, available on the RCOG site. By reading these leaflets the candidate is likely to get familiar with the kind of language to be used while counselling the patient.

Variations

The possible variations in this station are that there can be similar preoperative scenarios associated with several surgeries such as caesarean section, diagnostic laparoscopy, diagnostic hysteroscopy, tubal sterilisation, etc.

REFERENCES

1. Hall JA, Roter DL, Rand CS. Communication of affect between patient and physician. J Health Soc Behav. 1981;22(1):18-30.
2. Ha JF, Longnecker N. Doctor-patient communication: a review. Ochsner J. 2010;10(1):38-43.
3. Duffy FD, Gordon GH, Whelan G, et al. Assessing competence in communication and interpersonal skills: the Kalamazoo II report. Acad Med. 2004;79(6):495-507.
4. van Zanten M, Boulet JR, McKinley DW, et al. Assessing the communication and interpersonal skills of graduates of international medical schools as part of the United States Medical Licensing Exam (USMLE) Step 2 Clinical Skills (CS) Exam. Acad Med. 2007;82(10 Suppl):S65-S68.
5. Brédart A, Bouleuc C, Dolbeault S. Doctor-patient communication and satisfaction with care in oncology. Curr Opin Oncol. 2005;17(14):351-4.
6. Royal College of Obstetricians and Gynaecologists (RCOG). The Care of Women Requesting Induced Abortion. Evidence based Clinical Guideline Number 7. London: RCOG; 2011.
7. Harrison MR, Adzick NS, Estes JM, et al. A prospective study of the outcome for fetuses with diaphragmatic hernia. JAMA. 1994;271:382-4.
8. Bollmann R, Kalache K, Mau H, et al. Associated malformations and chromosomal defects in congenital diaphragmatic hernia. Fetal Diagn Ther. 1995;10:52-9.
9. McPherson EW, Ketterer DM, Salsburey DJ. Pallister-Killian and Fryns syndromes: nosology. Am J Med Genet. 1993;47:241-5.
10. Delvaux V, Moerman P, Fryns JP. Diaphragmatic hernia in the Coffin-Siris syndrome. Genet Couns. 1998;9:45-50.
11. Royal College of Obstetricians and Gynecologists. Amniocentesis and chorionic villus sampling. Green-top Guideline No. 8. London: RCOG; 2010.
12. Nuovo J, Melnikow J, Willan AR, et al. Treatment outcomes for squamous intraepithelial lesions. Int J Gynaecol Obstet. 2000;68(1):25-33.
13. Plante M, Renaud MC, Hoskins IA, et al. Vaginal radical trachelectomy: a valuable fertility-preserving option in the management of early-stage cervical cancer. A series of 50 pregnancies and review of the literature. Gynecol Oncol. 2005;98(1):3-10.
14. Shepherd JH, Spencer C, Herod J, et al. Radical vaginal trachelectomy as a fertility-sparing procedure in women with early-stage cervical cancer-cumulative pregnancy rate in a series of 123 women. BJOG. 2006;113(6):719-24.

15. DiSaia PJ, Creasman WT, Mannel RD, et al (Eds). Clinical Gynecologic Oncology, 9th edition. St Louis: Mosby; 2017.
16. Cancer Waiting Times Team. Cancer Waiting Times: A Guide (Version 9.0). Leeds: Cancer Waiting Times Team; 2015.
17. Improving Independent Complaints Advocacy in Health and Social Care: Background and Position Briefing. Healthwatch England. November 2013. Available from http://www.healthwatch.co.uk/sites/healthwatch.co.uk/files/complaints_advocacy.pdf [Accessed September 2017].
18. Elson CJ, Salim R, Potdar N, et al; on behalf of the Royal College of Obstetricians and gynaecologists. Diagnosis and management of ectopic pregnancy. BJOG. 2016;123: e15-e55.
19. Moskowitz DM, Klein JJ, Shander A, et al. Use of the Hemobag for modified ultrafiltration in a Jehovah's Witness patient undergoing cardiac surgery. J Extra Corpor Technol. 2006;38(3):265-70.
20. Issued by the Lord Chancellor. Mental Capacity Act, 2005. Code of Practice (2007) London: TSO.

6

Communication with Colleagues

INTRODUCTION

Since it is not possible for any doctor to work in complete isolation, communication with colleagues in health care forms an essential part of the everyday practice. Poor communication skills are the likely cause of most complaints, claims, and disciplinary actions in the medical practice. Failure of communication between doctors as well as the failure of communication between the patient and the doctor is likely to result in considerable risk to the patients.[1] A review of patient safety events in general practice in the year 2008 by Makeham et al. has shown that nearly 13% of reported errors are likely to occur as a result of communication failure. Of these, nearly 70% of the errors are related to interaction with the hospital or other health care professionals.[2] A review of paediatric care in 2007 by Hain et al. demonstrated that nearly 50% of the adverse outcomes were related to poor inter-professional interaction.[3] Poor communication between the multidisciplinary, interprofessional medical team is likely to increase the rates of surgical errors, endanger patient safety, and increase the rate of various complications as well as the overall rate of mortality and morbidity.[4-6]

The importance of communication skills for the doctors with their patients as well as with their colleagues is well established. While communication with the patients has been discussed in details in Chapter 5, communication skills with medical colleagues (both senior and junior) are discussed in details in this chapter.

In the MRCOG Part 3 examination, the candidates are expected to demonstrate their ability to express information to the medical colleagues concisely, in a logical and structured way. In these tasks, the candidate must be able to summarise their history, examination, and results of investigation, while focusing on the salient features. They should be able to present a clear and well-reasoned plan to their medical colleague. The candidate's ability to summarise and convey relevant information demonstrates their ability to think critically regarding what is important and the reason for communication of those facts. Communication tasks with medical colleagues in the part 3 examination may include an assessment of communication with colleagues in both verbal and written forms. Written tasks in the part 3 examination may involve tasks such as writing operation notes, preparing a letter to the GP, writing a referral to another specialty, and preparing a discharge summary or a prescription. The competent candidate should have clear, legible handwriting in the tasks involving writing. The candidates must therefore practice their writing prior to attempting the part 3 examination because they may have been in the practice of maintaining electronic records.

Communication between medical colleagues requires a different level of skills in comparison to the communication with patients. While communicating with the patients, the doctor must avoid the use of medical jargon. On the other hand, while communicating with the colleagues, it is important that the doctor uses medical terminology.

When communicating with each other, doctors tend to use medical terminology in their conversation to ensure that their communication is accurate and precise, and is not misinterpreted by their colleagues. However, while communicating with the junior colleague, the senior doctor must ensure that the junior colleagues understand what has been told to them. Therefore, while using medical terminology, the senior doctor must check to see whether the junior colleagues understand what they have been taught. During the MRCOG Part 3 examination, the situation is slightly different because the simulated junior colleagues are actors in the various candidate-simulated-trainee OSCE stations and therefore are unlikely to understand anatomical terms. Consequently, the candidate must preferably avoid the use of medical terminology or ask the simulated trainee whether they understand what is been told to them in case the candidate does use medical terminology.

MODES OF COMMUNICATION

The various reasons due to which the doctors may be required to communicate with their medical colleagues are described next.

Transfer of Information

Patient Handover

Since most junior doctors, consultants, nursing, and midwifery staff in the National Health Service (NHS) work in shift duties, there would be number of times during a 24-hour period when staff would be changing. In such situations, it is essential that the patient handover occurs to ensure that patient care continues flawlessly even though the workforce has changed. This implies that the doctors (especially senior trainees and consultants) need to develop the skills for communicating with their medical, nursing, and midwifery colleagues and safely take the patient handover, via the notes for both inpatients and outpatients. While taking the handover from the medical colleagues, a special training 5 (ST5) level candidate must note down the essential positive findings, relevant negative findings, and the important tasks, which still need to be completed in order to ensure an adequate, subsequent care plan for such patients.

The candidates must preferably use a structured system of communication for handover such as the SBAR tool (*Situation*, *Background*, *Assessment* and *Recommendations*). This tool helps in ensuring that no important information is missed while the information is being transferred. Candidates are expected to demonstrate their ability to convey information briefly and in a logical and structured manner.

Communication at handover is a core clinical skill, particularly on a labour ward, and is likely to be tested in the part 3 examination. Safe and efficient handover comprises of a list of patients, brief description of their clinical situation, investigations, which are done as well as those, which are awaited, and the tasks, which require to be completed. Handovers must also draw attention towards the high-risk patients who require review and who are at the risk of facing further deterioration in their clinical condition. While it is important to provide adequate amount of information at the time of handover, it is also important to develop the skill of being concise and simultaneously cover all the relevant issues related to the patient care so that the team taking handover can effortlessly continue with patient care. The handover process also evaluates the candidate's ability to triage and correctly prioritise their workload. The main problem the candidates are likely to face in the part 3 examination is that they have only 10 minutes to complete their handover, so they need to carefully manage their time. On such stations, the candidate must start telling the examiner first about the more complex patients, which require urgent attention, followed by those, which are relatively straightforward.

Maintaining checklists is a useful way for ensuring that there is complete transfer of information while referring a patient. Checklists can be used as memory aids or assimilated into the records or correspondence letters. This empowers the doctors to concentrate on more the complex tasks by reducing the amount of information they need to remember and process at one time.[7] When undertaking handovers, it is important to check that the information has been correctly understood by the person to whom the handover has been given. For this, a process of 'check-back' may be undertaken, where the health care professional receiving the handover repeats back the key points that they have understood.

Another method for reducing risk when passing care to a colleague includes the use of information technology systems to automate transfer of information and use of tracking systems for referrals, investigations, and follow-up.

Communication with the GP

The consultants and the senior trainees in the UK also need to communicate with their colleagues in primary care or GPs. Communication with colleagues must be concise, relevant, and to the point. Large pieces of information must be broken into more manageable pieces of information.

Communication with the Multidisciplinary Team

It is essential for the obstetrician and gynaecologist to be able to communicate appropriately with all the other health care professionals who form part of the multidisciplinary team taking care of the women with obstetric or gynaecological problems. This team includes not only doctors taking care of the women, but also nurses working in traditional roles, as well as nurses and midwives with clinical responsibilities of their own. For example, a gynaecological multidisciplinary team helps in linking gynaecologists with pathologists, radiologists, radiotherapists, oncologists, and specialist oncology nurses.

Midwives form an important component of the multidisciplinary team caring for an obstetric patient. The candidate must remember that in the UK, midwives are independent practitioners having the responsibility for caring for women with uncomplicated pregnancy. In fact, in the UK midwives entirely take care of a vast majority of pregnant women throughout their pregnancy and the postnatal period, without requiring any help from the medical team. Midwives help identify women, who develop complications during pregnancy and require transition to consultant-led care. Midwives are also important for identifying those women who are high-risk and require consultant-led care right from the beginning. Nevertheless, midwives would also provide considerable support to the high-risk women under consultant-led care. Therefore, it is essential for the doctor to be able to communicate with, and work in collaboration with the midwives. They should also have a clear understanding, regarding the tasks which are appropriate to be delegated to midwives or other members of the health care team (e.g. specialists nurses such as oncology nurses, diabetic nurses, gynaecological nurses, etc.; consultant midwives, etc.), the tasks they should undertake themselves and when to call for senior help. The specialist nurses, midwives, and consultant midwives with extended roles act as independent health care professionals in the UK providing direct care for patients working alongside doctors. To ensure patient safety, their work is guided by protocols and standard operating procedures. In cases where clinical situations fall outside these protocols (e.g. woman with complex mental health requirements, etc.), midwives and/or specialists nurses must refer the woman to the medical team. Communication-centred tasks in the part 3 examination are likely to assess the candidates' ability to work as part of the team and their leadership skills. The tasks may include situations where the candidate may have to deal with clinical disagreement with medical, nursing or midwifery colleagues. The candidate must also develop skills for sensitively dealing with behavioural issues.

Teaching Skills

One of the core duties of a doctor has been defined by the General Medical Council (GMC) as teaching the junior colleagues. Teaching a particular manoeuvre (e.g. for shoulder dystocia) or a practical skill (e.g. management of a case of post-partum haemorrhage), either in the form of a tutorial or doing some bedside teaching such as a case-based discussion may be assessed in the part 3 examination. The candidates attempting the MRCOG Part 3 examination are expected to be at ST5 level and would be entering the final phases of training before becoming a consultant. Therefore, they already have the responsibility of teaching the next generation of trainees in obstetrics and gynaecology. It is important that they understand not only the principles of adult learning, but are also acquainted with the best ways for demonstrating that knowledge. The candidate must communicate with their junior colleague in a clear, concise, and consistent manner, and simultaneously also show respect for them. They must ascertain that the learner has understood what they have been taught and would be able to adapt to it and apply that knowledge during their own training. The candidate is expected to understand all aspects of teaching, including the teaching of a practical skill, preparation of a teaching session, and the use of audio-visual aids and mannequins (dummy doll and dummy pelvis). The candidate should develop the necessary skills to ensure that the junior trainees are able to fully understand the topic of the teaching session in order to ensure appropriate patient safety and simultaneously also demonstrate their applied clinical knowledge. The candidate must intervene if patient safety is at risk. In the MRCOG Part 3 examination, the simulated trainee may be instructed to intentionally misunderstand a procedure or carry out a step of the procedure incorrectly to evaluate whether or not the candidate intervenes in between, without upsetting or discouraging the learner.

Teaching any skill can be broken down into a series of three steps as described next. These three steps can be considered as the best way for reinforcing the steps of a procedure in the learner's mind and promoting understanding.

Step 1: Demonstrating the Skill to the Trainee

The candidate must run through the steps of demonstration while explaining the trainee simultaneously what they are doing.

Step 2: The Trainee then Explains the Trainer What is to be Done

The candidate must ask the learner to explain the task back to him or her (the teacher), while the trainer is performing the procedure.

Step 3: Hands-on Training

Finally, the trainee must be given hands-on training and instructed to do the procedure themselves while explaining what they are doing.

However, all these steps must be finished within the stipulated time of 10 minutes. Therefore, time management remains the core principle behind the success in these kinds of stations. The competent candidate would also encourage learner to ask questions at the end of demonstration. The competent candidates would also be willing to repeat their instructions or give a logical explanation in response to the learner's questions. At the conclusion of the teaching session, the candidate must present an action plan for the simulated trainee demonstrating how they can improve and/or implement their new skills in practice.

Providing Feedback

Providing constructive feedback to the trainee remains the essence behind teaching a clinical skill to the trainee. This should preferably involve recognition and strengthening of the procedural steps, which have been performed well by the trainee. This should be then followed by the discussion of things, which could have been improved. The candidate must demonstrate the trainee how their technique can be improved, or modified to achieve a more successful outcome. In the end, they must summarise the good points again and make a plan for further development.

The candidate must avoid starting a discussion with criticism because this is likely to result in the development of a defensive attitude in the learner. This implies that the trainee may be unlikely to accept any constructive comments thereafter.

Writing Prescriptions

Ability to write prescriptions accurately and legibly tests both candidate's written communication skills and patient safety. It is really important for the candidate attempting the part 3 examination to be able to write accurate prescriptions. In case, the candidate is not familiar with the style of prescription charts used in the NHS, some actually useful information regarding the prescription charts is available on the website of the Academy of Medical Royal Colleges (http://www.aomrc.org.uk/). There is a strong emphasis in the NHS that antibiotics should be prescribed under proper supervision. Therefore, any prescription for antibiotics should have a stop date. The prescriptions should also have a date when microbial sensitivities would be checked to ensure that the most appropriate drug is being used.

Writing clinic letters and referral letters to other specialties also involves special skills. The letter to the clinic should not contain the exact information, which is mentioned in the referral letter. In fact, it should highlight any salient fact, which the clinician noted at the time of consultation or examination. The clinician must also highlight the results of any investigations along with a clear plan for management and/or follow-up. If the letter is written for the GP, the task which the GP is required to do, e.g. prescribing medication or checking coil threads, needs to be clearly mentioned in the body of the letter. Though the MRCOG examination does not test English language, candidates should be familiar with the use of grammar, punctuation, and spellings to ensure that the messages in the letter are clear.

IDENTIFYING RISKS

The reasons why doctors may not communicate sufficient information to their colleagues about patients under their care include the following:

- *Pressures of time*: Changes in working patterns and the resultant increase in shift work and cross cover in the NHS implies that a large number of doctors and health care professionals may be involved in a patient's care. This has increased the risk of failures in communication at the time of passing care

between doctors during a referral or a handover, thereby increasing the possibility that patient information may not be properly shared. As a result, abnormal results of the investigation may be missed, treatments may be inadequately monitored, or important comorbidities may not be taken into account. All these factors may put the patient at an increased risk of harm. Good documentation of patient records helps in dealing with this risk.
- Difficulty in accessing colleagues.
- Difficult relationships with the colleagues.

Disagreements with Colleagues

Differences of opinion between the medical doctors pose a detrimental risk for the patient. Deviations in opinion may occur over several issues such as diagnosis, treatment, management, interpretation of investigations, resource allocation, and end of life issues.

When trying to resolve a disagreement with a colleague, the doctors must keep the following important principles in their mind:[8]
- They have an obligation to act in the patient's best interests
- They must work in collaboration with their colleagues, treating them with respect and dignity. They must also respect their skills and contributions.

OSCE STATION 1: TRAINING A JUNIOR COLLEAGUE ON BREECH VAGINAL DELIVERY

Candidate's Instructions

You have been asked by the department's tutor to teach the fourth-year medical student attached to your department about conducting a breech vaginal delivery.

A doll and a mannequin have been provided to help you demonstrate this obstetric technique. The task is for 12 minutes (inclusive of 2 minutes of reading time). You have 10 minutes to teach the simulated trainee about conducting a breech vaginal delivery. You shall be awarded marks for the following tasks:

Candidate's tasks:
- Explain the candidate the method of conducting a breech vaginal delivery
- Explain the various techniques for delivering the after-coming head of the breech
- Explain the various techniques for delivering the legs in case of breech presentation.

These tasks cover the domains as discussed next.

Core Clinical Skills Domains

Core clinical skills domains tested:
- Patient safety
- Communication with colleagues
- Application of knowledge.

Module Tested

The modules tested in this station are Module 1 or 'Teaching', Module 6 or 'Management of Labour', and Module 7 or 'Management of Delivery'.

Role-player's Brief

- You are Emma Bond, a fourth-year medical student and this is your first undergraduate posting in obstetrics and gynaecology.
- You spent some time on the labour ward last night and the woman whom you were observing had breech presentation. You found the entire procedure of breech vaginal delivery very fascinating and you would want to yourself conduct a breech vaginal delivery. You explained this to your tutor, who has arranged one of the registrars to teach you today about breech vaginal delivery.
- The candidate is supposed to talk to you about the method of conducting a breech vaginal delivery and explain you various manoeuvres especially those associated with the delivery of after-coming head of the breech as well as the delivery of baby's legs.

Prompt Questions

If he or she does not cover the following points, then you should ask:
- 'When do I give an episiotomy?'
- 'What do I do if the baby's head cannot be delivered by either Burn's Marshall or Mauriceau–Smellie–Veit Manoeuvre?'
- What do I do if the baby's buttocks have delivered, but the legs are stuck up?'

EXAMINER'S INSTRUCTIONS AND STRUCTURED MARK SHEET

The examiner will mark the candidate on the basis of various tasks, which are allotted to the candidate. Out of a total score of 20, the examiner can award a maximum of 18 marks, which are distributed between various candidate tasks as shown next. The role-player can award a maximum of 2 marks to the candidate. Each candidate task must be globally scored by the examiner.

The examiners need to familiarise themselves with the candidate's instructions.

Method for Conducting a Breech Vaginal Delivery

- Before explaining the procedure of breech vaginal delivery, the candidate spends few minutes in explaining why breech vaginal delivery is preferred over caesarean delivery in this case.
- Places the mannequin in lithotomy position and brings the buttocks to the end of the bed or table.
- Once the buttocks have entered the vagina and the cervix is fully dilated, the woman must be advised to bear down with the contractions, thereby allowing the breech to distend the perineum.

- Episiotomy may be performed, if the perineum appears very tight.
- The candidate must instruct the role-player to adopt a 'no-touch policy/ hands off the breech policy' until the buttocks and lower back deliver till the level of umbilicus. At this point the baby's shoulder blades can be seen.[9]
- The role-player can be instructed to place their fingers on the sacrum and bony pelvis to guide the rotation of the baby.
- The candidate must explain the role-player that sometimes they may have to make use of manoeuvres like Pinard's manoeuvre and groin traction if the legs have not delivered spontaneously.
- The candidate should advise the role-player to be extremely careful and gently hold the baby by wrapping it in a clean cloth in such a way that the baby's trunk is present anteriorly. This will allow the foetal head to enter the pelvis in occipitoanterior position.
- The baby must be held by the hips and not by the flanks or abdomen as this may cause kidney or liver damage. Candidate must instruct the role-player that at no point, they must try to pull the baby out, rather the patient must be encouraged to push down.
- In order to avoid compression on the umbilical cord, it should be moved to one side, preferably in the sacral bay.
- In case of extended breech, the role-player can be instructed to flex the baby's knee to deliver them.
- The role-player must be instructed to help deliver the arms by flexing them over the baby's chest.
- Following the delivery of rest of the body, the role-player must allow the baby to hang by its weight.
- Candidate first demonstrates the various steps and then allows the role-player to demonstrate them initially by assisting the role-player, followed later by just observing them.

Marking Scheme

0	1	2	3	4
Fail	Borderline		Pass	

Various Techniques for Delivering the after-coming Head of the Breech

Candidate demonstrates delivery of after-coming head of the breech using any of the three techniques: Burns–Marshall technique, Mauriceau–Smellie–Veit manoeuvre, and forceps.

Burns–Marshall Technique

- Demonstrates to let the baby hang unsupported from the mother's vulva, once the shoulders and both the arms of the baby have delivered, to encourage flexion of the foetal head (Fig. 6.1A).
- Application of the suprapubic pressure in downward and backward direction by the assistant in order to encourage further flexion of the baby's head.

- Efforts must be made by the candidate to deliver the baby's head by grasping the foetal ankles with the finger of right hand between the two as soon as the nape of baby's neck appears. Then the trunk is swung up forming a wide arc of the circle, while maintaining continuous traction when doing this (Fig. 6.1B).
- Candidate demonstrates the use of left hand to provide pelvic support and to clear the perineum off successively from the baby's face and brow as the baby's head emerges out.

Mauriceau–Smellie–Veit Manoeuvre

- Candidate places the baby face down with the length of the baby's body over his or her supinated left forearm and hand.
- The candidate then demonstrates placing his or her first (index) and second finger (middle finger) of their left hand on the baby's cheekbones and the thumb over the baby's chin. This helps in facilitating flexion of the foetal head.
- The candidate advises the role-player that placing a finger inside the infant's mouth must not be done because it is supposed to stimulate the vagal reflex.
- Simultaneous application of suprapubic pressure by an assistant helps in keeping the baby's head flexed.
- The candidate uses his or her right hand for grasping the baby's shoulders. The little finger and the ring finger of the candidate's right hand are placed over the baby's right shoulder, the index finger over the baby's left shoulder,

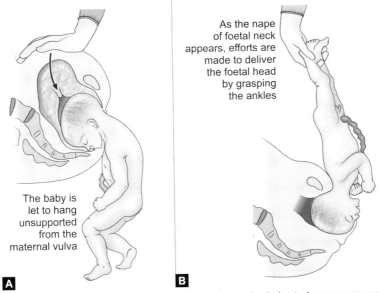

As the nape of foetal neck appears, efforts are made to deliver the foetal head by grasping the ankles

The baby is let to hang unsupported from the maternal vulva

A   **B**

Figs. 6.1A and B: Burns Marshall technique. (A) Baby is let to hang unsupported from the maternal vulva; (B) As the nape of foetal neck appears, efforts are made to deliver the foetal head by grasping the foetal ankles and swinging the trunk up by forming a wide arc of circle.

and the middle finger over the baby's suboccipital region (Figs. 6.2A to C). With the fingers of right hand in this position, the baby's head is flexed towards the chest. At the same time left hand is used for applying downward pressure on the jaw to bring the baby's head down until the hairline is visible.

- Thereafter the baby's trunk is carried in upwards and forwards direction towards the maternal abdomen, till the baby's mouth, nose and brow, and lastly the vertex and occiput have been released.
- The candidate uses both the arms in synchronisation to exert gentle downwards traction simultaneously both on the foetal neck and maxilla.
- While performing the Mauriceau–Smellie–Veit manoeuvre, the candidate must instruct the role-player to avoid pulling on the jaw and the importance of keeping the baby's head flexed with the application of malar pressure.

Delivery of after-coming Head Using Forceps

- Application of forceps (Fig. 6.3) is the technique of choice to ensure safe delivery of baby's head because it provides protection to the foetal head from sudden forces of compression and decompression.

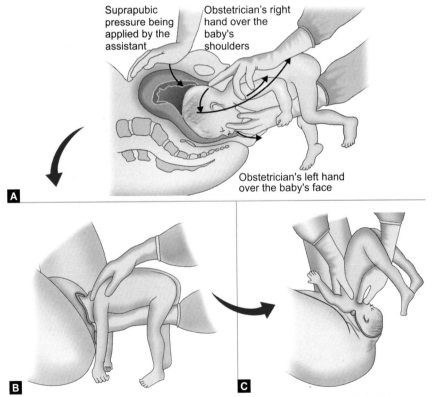

Figs. 6.2A to C: Mauriceau–Smellie–Veit manoeuvre. (A) The baby is laid flat over the obstetrician's forearm with the fingers of left hand over the baby's face and right hand over the occiput; (B) The baby's head is gradually flexed; (C) The baby's trunk is carried upwards and forwards to deliver the foetal head.

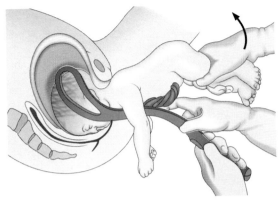

Fig. 6.3: Delivery of after-coming head of the breech using forceps.

- Use of forceps helps in better maintenance of flexion of foetal head and helps in transmitting the force to the foetal head rather than the neck. This helps in reducing the risk of foetal injuries. Furthermore, flexion of foetal head helps in reducing the diameter of foetal head, thereby aiding descent.
- Ordinary forceps or Piper's forceps (specially designed forceps with absent pelvic curve) or divergent Laufe's forceps can be used.
- While the candidate is applying forceps, they must instruct the role-player to wrap the baby's body in a cloth or towel and ask the assistant to hold it on one side. Suspension of the baby in a towel prior to application of forceps helps in effectively holding the baby's body and keeping the arms out of the way.
- At the time of application of forceps, the assistant must hold the infant's body at or just above the horizontal plane. Assistant must be instructed not to hold the foetal body higher than this plane because hyperextension of foetal neck can cause injuries such as dislocation of cervical spine, bleeding in the venous plexus around the cervical spine, and sometimes even quadriplegia.
- The candidate must instruct the role-player to first apply left blade of the forceps followed by the right blade and then lock the handles.
- The forceps are used for both flexing and delivering the baby's head. During the initial descent of foetal head, foetal body must remain in horizontal plane. Once the chin and mouth are visible over the perineum, the forceps and the body and legs of the foetus are raised to complete delivery.
- The candidate must explain to the role-player to slowly deliver the foetal head over 1 minute in order to avoid sudden compression or decompression of foetal head, which may be a cause for intracranial haemorrhage.

Marking Scheme

0	1	2	3	4
Fail	Borderline		Pass	

(The examiner needs to adjust the marks if role-player has to prompt)

Delivery of the Baby's Legs

If the baby's buttocks and hip do not deliver by themselves, the candidate demonstrates the use of simple manoeuvres including groin traction or Pinard's manoeuvre to the role-player for delivering the legs.

Groin Traction

- The candidate must teach the role-player about two types of groin traction: single groin traction and double groin traction.
- In single groin traction, the candidate must instruct the role-player to hook the index finger of one hand in the baby's groin fold and exert traction towards the foetal trunk rather than towards the foetal femur, in accordance with the uterine contractions.
- In double groin traction, the candidate must instruct the role-player to hook the index fingers of both the hands in the baby's groin folds and then apply traction (Fig. 6.4).

Pinard's Manoeuvre

- In this manoeuvre, candidate instructs the role-player to exert pressure against the inner aspect of the baby's knee (popliteal fossa), with help of the middle and index fingers of the right hand (Fig. 6.5A).
- As the pressure is applied, the knee gets flexed and abducted. This causes the lower leg to move downwards, which the candidate must sweep medially and gently pull out of the vagina (Figs. 6.5B and C).

Marking Scheme

0	1	2	3	4
Fail	Borderline		Pass	

(The examiner needs to adjust the marks if role-player has to prompt)

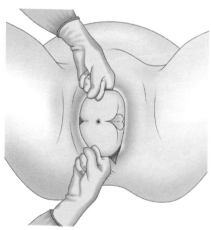

Fig. 6.4: Application of groin traction.

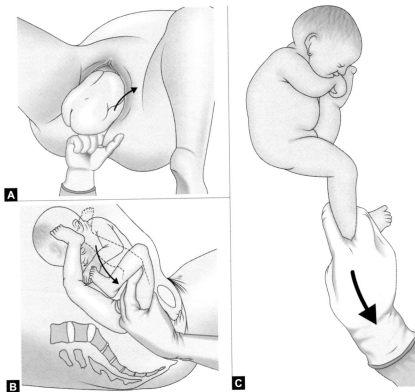

Figs. 6.5A to C: Pinard's manoeuvre. (A) Pressure is exerted against the popliteal fossa; (B) Due to application of pressure, the foetal knee gets flexed and abducted; (C) As the foetal leg moves downwards, it is pulled out by the clinician.

Demonstrates the procedure adequately.

0	1	2
Fail	Borderline	Pass

Takes the role-player through the procedure.

0	1	2
Fail	Borderline	Pass

Allows role-player to demonstrate what he or she has been taught.

0	1	2
Fail	Borderline	Pass

Role-player's Score

The role-player can award a maximum of 2 marks to the candidate.

Marking Scheme

0	1	2
No confidence in being able to deal with breech vaginal delivery	Reasonably confident in being able to deal with breech vaginal delivery	Fully confident in being able to deal with breech vaginal delivery

Total score: /20

DISCUSSION

Issues

With such kinds of stations, the candidates are able to demonstrate their teaching skills to the junior colleagues. The candidate must remember to demonstrate various manoeuvres to the role-player in a step-by-step manner. They must also keep asking the role-player if they are understanding the various steps or not. They should allow the role-players to go through the various steps themselves and to demonstrate each step (as they have been taught) on the mannequin.

Pitfalls

Not asking the role-players if they had been able to understand various steps of the procedure can be considered as a potential mistake. Also not allowing the role-players to demonstrate each step as they had been taught can be considered as a serious mistake.

Variations

Variations in this kind of station could include teaching the junior colleagues regarding various techniques and manoeuvres related to several conditions, e.g. management of a case with shoulder dystocia, technique of external cephalic version, conducting a normal vaginal delivery, application of forceps, vacuum, etc.

OSCE STATION 2: TEACHING A JUNIOR COLLEAGUE METHOD OF TAKING CONSENT

Candidate's Instructions

You are an ST5 and a junior trainee (second foundation year) has recently joined your department. The trainee will be required to take consent for an emergency laparotomy from the patient, Mrs Lucy brown with ruptured ectopic pregnancy. You are getting ready for the laparotomy when you notice that this trainee has already filled in the consent form for this patient (Fig. 6.6). The task is for 12 minutes (inclusive of 2 minutes of reading time). You have 10 minutes

Patient Identifier/Label

Name: Lucy Brown

DOB: 06/09/1986

Name of proposed procedure of course of treatment (include brief explanation if medical term not clear)

Emergency laparotomy (opening up the abdominal cavity for dealing with ruptured ectopic pregnancy)

Statement of the health professional (to be filled in by health professional with appropriate knowledge of proposed procedure as specified in consent policy)

I have explained the procedure to the patient. In particular, I have explained.

The intended benefits

The tube containing the ectopic pregnancy has ruptured resulting in internal haemorrhage. A cut would be given in the abdomen to visualise and repair the ruptured tube. If required the ruptured tube would be removed

Serious or frequently occurring risks Haemorrhage, requirement for blood transfusion or requirement for hysterectomy (rarely), recurrent ectopic, poor fertility outcome in subsequent pregnancies.

Any Extra procedures which may become necessary during the procedure

☑ Blood transfusion

☐ Other Procedure (Please specify)

I have also discussed what the procedure is likely to involve, the benefits and risk of any available alternative treatments (including no treatment) and any particular concerns of this patient.

☑ The following leaflets has been provided Ectopic pregnancy

The procedure will involve:

☑ General and/or regional anesthesia ☐ local anesthesia ☐ Sedation

Signed [signature] Date 6/4/17

Name (PRINT) ASHLEY BROWN Job title FY2 ObGYN

Contact Details (if patient wishes to discuss options later) Mrs Perkins Secretary Extension 4920 Labour ward extension 4433

Statement of Interpreter (where appropriate) Not required

I have interpreted the above information to the patient in a way in which I believe s/he can understand

Signed Date

Name (PRINT)

TOP COPY accepted by the patient (Yes)/No (please ring)

Fig. 6.6: Consent form as filled by the simulated trainee.

to counsel the trainee about the situation. You shall be awarded marks for the following tasks:

Candidate's tasks:

- Review the consent form with the junior doctor and provide feedback
- Explain the principles of obtaining valid consent
- Support the trainee in their ongoing education.

These tasks cover the domains as discussed next.

Core Clinical Skills Domains

Core clinical skills domains tested:

- Patient safety
- Communication with patients
- Communication with colleagues
- Application of knowledge.

Module Tested

The modules tested in this station are Module 1 or 'Teaching' and Module 2 or 'Surgical Skills'.

Role-player's Brief

You are Ashley Brown, a junior trainee in obstetrics 1 year after qualification (FY2) who has just joined the department on rotation. As part of your duties, you will have to take consent for an emergency laparotomy in case of ruptured ectopic pregnancy.

You were asked by the nursing staff to obtain consent from a woman, who had been admitted with the diagnosis of ectopic pregnancy. Few minutes ago, she collapsed and the registrar in your unit is expecting this due to rupture of the ectopic pregnancy. As a result, she is posted for an emergency laparotomy for which you have been asked to take consent. The nursing staff had also briefly explained to you about the seriousness of the event and why it is an emergency situation.

You were trained by the midwife a day ago to take consent in case of an elective caesarean section. You have used that knowledge as well as what you remember being taught about consent in the days of your medical school. You always did well at medical school, but there was not much teaching about taking consent during your obstetric module. You know about the implications and consequences of a ruptured ectopic pregnancy. Otherwise, you are a self-confident individual and you believe you have sufficient medical knowledge. You take advice from your colleagues only if you find what they are saying is convincing enough.

Prompt Questions

- Should I need to tell the patient about the risks, which are really rare?
- How is it possible for me to fit everything in the consent form?
- If I had included all the risks, would not the patient have refused the procedure?

EXAMINER'S INSTRUCTIONS AND STRUCTURED MARK SHEET

The examiner will mark the candidate on the basis of various tasks, which are allotted to the candidate. Out of a total score of 20, the examiner can award a maximum of 18 marks, which are distributed between various candidate tasks as shown next. The role-player can award a maximum of 2 marks to the candidate. Each candidate task must be globally scored by the examiner.

Reviewing the Consent Form with the Junior Doctor

- The candidate needs to highlight the good points in the way consent was documented by the role-player.
- Another important element, which the candidate must highlight to the role-player, is that they need to be properly trained prior to taking consent. The competent candidate must guarantee that the trainees precisely understand the significance of a ruptured ectopic pregnancy and the requirement of an emergency laparotomy before they start taking consent. This would help in demonstrating the candidate's concern about the patient safety.
- The simulated trainee or role-player needs to understand that they are required to know about the benefits and risk of the procedure before they can communicate this to the patient.
- While considering information gathering, the competent candidate shall try to find out what the junior trainee understands, what their concerns are, and then ensure that these are addressed in an appropriate manner.
- The competent candidate will guarantee that the role-player has clearly grasped the instructions given to him. They need to ascertain that role-player has understood the implications of what he or she has been taught. He or she should also be able to comprehend it and can repeat it when asked to mention the relevant points. This would help to ensure the learning has been implanted in the role-player's mind.
- Feedback should be given objectively and without undermining the junior trainee.

Providing Appropriate Feedback

- Praising the role-player regarding the use of legible writing and avoiding the use of abbreviations and medical jargon.
- The candidate must also tactfully outline the mistakes, which the simulated trainee has made, and correct mistakes in the consent. However, this must be done in way that the role-player does not get discouraged.
- The candidate shall provide beneficial feedback to the trainee regarding how they can improve their approach for taking consent.

Marking Scheme

0	1	2	3	4	5	6
Fail		Borderline		Pass		

Explaining the Principles of Obtaining Valid Consent[10,11]

- Assessment of mental capacity; the person giving consent must have the capacity to make the decision.
- Consent must be voluntary and informed.

- Permission must be taken after providing sufficient accurate information.
- A consent becomes invalid if the patient does not know what the intervention involves and that they have a right to refuse.
- Risks and alternatives to operation must be documented.
- Use of medical abbreviations and medical jargon should be avoided as far as possible.
- Consent should be taken by someone who can either undertake the procedure or who has been trained to take consent for that particular procedure.
- Role-player should not take consent until they are able to discuss the procedure and alternatives.
- Family members, including a spouse, do not have the right to know about confidential information regarding a patient unless she has given consent. This includes issues relating to contraception, care in pregnancy, and termination of pregnancy.

Marking Scheme

0	1	2	3	4	5	6
Fail		Borderline		Pass		

Supporting the Trainees in their ongoing Education

- The candidate must encourage reflection and self-directed learning in the simulated trainee.
- They should also tell the trainee about other resources such as hospital policies, RCOG guidelines, the GMC, or the Medical Defence Organisations, etc., from where they can further build up their knowledge related to taking consent from the patient.

Marking Scheme

0	1	2	3	4	5	6
Fail		Borderline		Pass		

Role-player's Score

The role-player can award a maximum of 2 marks to the candidate.

Marking Scheme

0	1	2
Role-player never wants to see candidate again	Role-player prepared to see candidate again	Role-player happy to see candidate again

Total score: /20

DISCUSSION

Issues

The ability to take an informed consent is an essential skill, which is likely to be tested in the MRCOG Part 3 examination. This question provides an opportunity to the examiner for assessing both communications with colleagues and communication with patients. While teaching the role-player about communicating with patients, a competent candidate would guarantee that the role-player writes the information on the consent form in such a way that even a non-medically qualified patient would be able to understand it.

It is essential for the candidate to adequately understand the principles of mental capacity as defined in both the Mental Capacity Act. Assessment of the patient's mental capacity involves the evaluation of her ability to understand, retain, and communicate the information after weighing the balance between the risks and benefits of the procedure. The patient must be provided with sufficient information to help her make a decision. Also, the patient must be able to give her consent freely. She should not be pressurized in any way for making her decision.

They also need to understand the principles of Fraser guidelines or Gillick's competency in relation to the adolescent girls (aged 13–18 years) looking for contraceptive advice or termination of pregnancy. There may be an OSCE station having a scenario where a teenager girl is asking for termination of pregnancy or advice regarding contraception. A candidate at ST5 level is required to be able to explain to the patients and their relatives, the disease conditions from which the patients are suffering, discuss the required investigations and treatment options and eventually obtain informed consent from them. Communication with patients in the practice of obstetrics and gynaecology requires a special level of skills, enabling the candidate to perform in highly stressful situations. They should also be able to inform, engage, negotiate, and enable shared decision-making.

Pitfalls

Some of the likely mistakes, which the candidates are likely to commit, include the following:
- Forgetting to introduce themselves and explaining their task to the role-player.
- Not listening to the junior colleagues or disrespecting their views.
- Insulting or undermining the junior colleague.
- Failing to ascertain from the simulated trainee that they understand the benefits and risk of the procedure before they can communicate this to the patient and subsequently take consent.

Variations

The stations related to teaching could be aimed at teaching a junior colleague about the principles related to taking consent for a major procedure (e.g. caesarean delivery, hysterectomy, laparotomy, etc.) or taking consent for a minor procedure (e.g. laparoscopy, hysteroscopy, suction curettage, taking endometrial biopsy, etc.). Variations in such kind of stations can be made by checking the candidate's ability to build relationships with their patients in a very short space of time when patients are often at their most stressed and most vulnerable state, for example, foetal distress requiring a category one caesarean section, stillbirth or a situation which is less stressful (e.g. taking consent for an elective caesarean delivery).

There could be a station where an adolescent girl asks for advise related to contraception.

OSCE STATION 3: DELIVERY USING FORCEPS

Candidate's Instructions

As the ST5 on call for obstetrics and gynaecology, you have just delivered the patient Alice Brown using forceps. The reason for application of forceps was that the baby was under distress. A junior colleague (ST1), who was watching you, wants to learn the procedure from you. She has no prior experience about the procedure. You have 10 minutes to demonstrate how you would teach the technique of forceps delivery in a case such as this to a junior colleague who has no prior experience about the procedure. Familiarise yourself with the candidate's instructions and simulated junior doctor's or role-player's instructions. Plan your approach to the task together.

The task is for 12 minutes (inclusive of 2 minutes of reading time). You have 10 minutes to teach the technique of forceps delivery to the simulated trainee. You shall be awarded marks for the following tasks:

Candidate's tasks:
- Communication with colleague
- Patient safety
- Application of knowledge.

These tasks cover the domains as discussed next.

Core Clinical Skills Domains

Core clinical skills domains tested:
- Patient safety
- Communication with colleagues
- Application of knowledge.

Module Tested

The modules tested in this station are Module 1 or 'Teaching' and Module 7 or 'Management of Delivery'.

Role-player's Brief

You are a junior doctor (ST1) with no prior experience of delivering a baby by forceps. You have asked the ST5 doctor (Registrar) on call with you today to teach you the procedure. You had been observing the doctor deliver a patient with foetal distress using forceps. The ST5 doctor must explain the procedure to you in a clear and logical manner and allow you to handle the equipment and practise its use.

Prompt Questions

- What parameters do I need to check before application of forceps?
- In what direction should I apply pressure while delivering the baby?
- Can I do the procedure myself using the doll and the dummy pelvis?

EXAMINER'S INSTRUCTIONS AND STRUCTURED MARK SHEET

The examiner will mark the candidate on the basis of various tasks, which are allotted to the candidate. Out of a total score of 20, the examiner can award a maximum of 18 marks, which are distributed between various candidate tasks as shown next. The role-player can award a maximum of 2 marks to the candidate. Each candidate task must be globally scored by the examiner.

Communication with Colleagues

- Follows a logical approach, correctly explains the sequence of events.
- Provides clear explanation of purpose and scope of the teaching session.
- The candidate emphasises to the role-player the requirement to introduce herself to the mum and keep the mother informed throughout the delivery.
- Asking the simulated junior doctor if they understand what has been explained to them.
- Candidate explains the meaning of technical terms used by them to the simulated trainee.
- The candidate must demonstrate the functioning of the equipment, including application of lubricant, correct application of the forceps to the foetal head, and correct application of traction.[12]
- Demonstrates the technique to the role-player and asks them to repeat the steps and helps in correcting their technique.
- A competent candidate would also spend a few seconds to explain why application of forceps is the correct choice of instrument in the given case.
- If a dummy pelvis and a baby doll are available on the station, then teach the simulated trainee using those.
- Also, gives the simulated trainee a chance to try his hand on the available equipment and encourages the trainee to be hands-on.

Marking Scheme

0	1	2	3	4	5	6
Fail		Borderline		Pass		

Patient Safety

- Taking an informed consent is essential prior to the procedure. The candidate must explain the role-player the method for obtaining verbal consent in case of forceps delivery. For an instrumental delivery in the delivery suite, verbal consent is sufficient in the majority of cases. However, in case of patients undergoing trial of vaginal delivery in an operation theatre, it is important to take written consent because such patients are at a high risk of requiring caesarean delivery.
- Patients need to understand what is being done to them, so the competent candidate must emphasise to the simulated trainee, the requirement for talking to the patient while conducting instrumental delivery. Simultaneously, the simulated trainee must comfort the patients, tell them what is being done and advise them when to 'push', 'pant' or rest as required. The simulated trainee must ask the mother to push before the crowning of the head occurs and to pant when crowning of the head occurs.
- Demonstrates to the role-player, how to correctly position the patient.
- Demonstrates the requirement for cleaning, draping, and catheterising the patient prior to the application of forceps.
- Explains the requirement for an abdominal as well as a vaginal examination.
- The competent candidate would advise the role-player to check for complete cervical dilatation and effacement and other prerequisites prior to the application of forceps.[13] They would also demonstrate to the simulated trainee to check for the position and station of foetal head prior to application.
- The candidate will teach how to deliver the baby safely by applying traction in the correct direction (Figs. 6.7A to C).[14]
- The competent candidate would help the simulated trainee to understand when an episiotomy is indicated in order to minimise the risk of a third- or fourth-degree tear. A competent candidate would also explain the requirement for prior perineal infiltration with local anaesthetic in case of an episiotomy.[15]
- The candidate must advise the simulated trainee to check for a nuchal cord and to allow restitution of the baby's head before delivering the body with the next contraction.
- They would then also explain the requirement to deliver the placenta.
- Following the delivery of the baby and the placenta, the perineum and vagina must be assessed for presence of any lacerations or tears. If any tear or episiotomy is present, it must be appropriately repaired. This must be clearly documented in the patient's notes.
- The candidates must also specify to the role-player when to abandon the procedure and proceed for a caesarean delivery (no descent even after three pulls).
- Other two important features of patient safety, which a competent candidate would not forget to explain the simulated trainee, are to estimate the amount of blood loss and to perform a swab as well as a needle count, both at the beginning and at the end of the procedure.

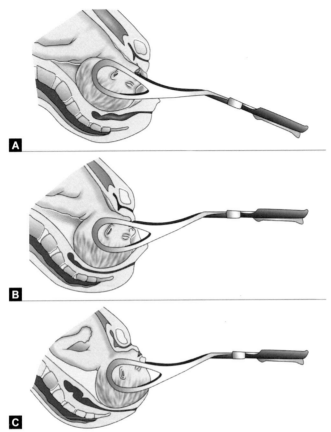

Figs. 6.7A to C: Directions of application of traction in case of forceps delivery. (A) Locking of forceps. Beginning traction in the axis of the birth canal; (B) Horizontal traction; (C) Delivery by flexion of the head.

Marking Scheme

0	1	2	3	4	5	6
Fail		Borderline		Pass		

Application of Knowledge

- Checks knowledge of the trainee before demonstrating the procedure to them.
- Explains the various prerequisites to be checked before applying forceps.
- Describes the correct technique of vaginal examination (using two fingers, rather than the whole hand) prior to the application of forceps.
- Correctly explains technical terms such as caput, moulding, occipitoanterior position, and station of the foetal head.
- Specifies the method of applying both the branches of the forceps in order to grip the foetal head.

- Describes the manner in which traction should be applied in the correct direction to deliver the baby's head.
- Also describes the amount of traction which must be applied.
- Specifies clear details while teaching the role-player about the method of administering an episiotomy.

Marking Scheme

0	1	2	3	4	5	6
Fail		Borderline		Pass		

Role-player's Score

The role-player can award a maximum of 2 marks to the candidate.

Marking Scheme

0	1	2
Role-player never wants to see candidate again	Role-player prepared to see candidate again	Role-player happy to see candidate again

Total score: /20

DISCUSSION

Assessing the skill of instrumental delivery (vacuum or forceps) should be straightforward for candidates attempting part 3 examination as this method of delivery is common in everyday use on the labour ward. The main purpose of this task is not only to assess the ability to carry out an instrumental delivery, but to evaluate candidate's deeper skills such as teaching. Teaching is an essential clinical skill, which has been defined by both the Part 2 MRCOG curriculum and by the GMC in Good Medical Practice Guidelines.

In order to be able to teach a skill to a junior colleague, the teacher must be competent in that skill and be at the top of Miller's triangle (Fig. 6.8). One must also remember that the word 'doctor' is an academic title derived from the Latin word of the same spelling and significance, meaning 'to teach'.[16] Passing on one's clinical skills form an essential aspect of the Hippocratic Oath.

Issues

The passing standard for such kind of tasks is high because such kind of clinical scenarios are commonly encountered in routine everyday situations. Also a candidate at ST5 level is likely to have mastered the technique of instrumental delivery (either forceps or ventouse) at a much earlier stage before reaching the ST5 level. Therefore, errors in these techniques are unacceptable and a severe cause for concern.

Not only is this station testing the candidate's skills to communicate with colleagues, it is also testing their interpersonal skills, an ability to provide

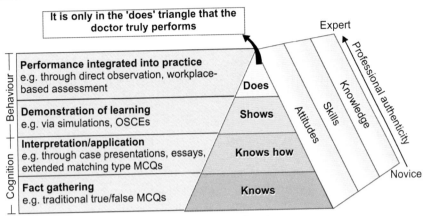

Fig. 6.8: Miller's triangle.

Source: Miller GE. The assessment of clinical skills/competence/performance. Acad Med. 1990;65(9):63-7. Adapted by Dr Mehay and Dr R Burns, UK (Jan 2009).

leadership in a teaching situation, an awareness of patient safety and, demonstration of applied clinical knowledge. Besides demonstrating how to do the procedure, the candidate must also tell the role-player regarding when to do or when not to do a procedure. In order to explain the procedure to the patient, the candidate should preferably break down the procedure into its component parts and explain it in a logical manner. While the patients must remain a doctor's first priority, building a rapport and passing on the clinical skills to junior colleagues are equally important. Junior colleagues must be respected and dealt with in a kind and supportive manner.

Though this is a straightforward task and there are no hidden tricks or catches in this station, it is completely possible that the simulated trainee may have been trained to do something incorrectly which may put a patient in danger. It is essential for the candidate to mediate in such situations and prevent harm without discouraging or embarrassing the trainee. Under no situation it is acceptable for the candidate to shout at the junior colleague or trainee.

Pitfalls

This station is not just assessing the candidate's ability to carry out an instrumental delivery, it also tests candidate's deeper skills, such as teaching. Failing to concentrate on demonstrating the teaching skills and just concentrating on the demonstration of skills for conducting an instrumental delivery can be considered as an important mistake in such kind of stations. The candidate must not describe the forceps delivery as a painful and traumatising procedure to the role-player.

An important skill for the candidates attempting the part 3 examination is to remain focused and specific. Another significant mistake would be to let the station move on to a discussion about a different topic such as shoulder dystocia, repair of third-degree tears or retained placenta. The candidates must carefully follow the instructions provided to them. The instructions in this station very clearly state that the technique of taking forceps delivery must be taught to the role-player. Therefore the candidate must stick to this.

Variations

While preparing for MRCOG Part 3 examination the candidates must practice with their exam buddy, imagining them to be a simulated trainee. They must practice by teaching them common skills encountered in clinical practice, which they are required to pass on to their junior colleagues. Some of these include method of conducting an instrumental delivery (both forceps and vacuum), manoeuvres used for the management of shoulder dystocia, breech presentation, method of repair of a third- or fourth-degree perineal repair, management of retained placenta, etc.

OSCE STATION 4: COMMUNICATION WITH THE SENIOR AND ANAESTHETIC COLLEAGUES BASED ON THE REQUIREMENTS (A POST-OPERATIVE PATIENT IN SHOCK)

Candidate's Instructions

You are the ST5 registrar posted in the post-operative ward. You are called by the nurse in charge of the post-operative ward to see Mrs Dorothy Wilde, a 53-year-old woman, who is noted to have a BP of 85/50 mmHg, a pulse of 123 beats/min, and poor urinary output. She underwent a vaginal hysterectomy for third-degree uterine prolapse 24 hours back.

The task is for 12 minutes (inclusive of 2 minutes of reading time). This task is a four-part structured discussion with the examiner. You have 10 minutes to answer the examiner's questions. You shall be awarded marks for the following tasks:

Candidate's tasks:

- What clinical features are indicative of shock in this case?
- What are the most likely causes of her shock?
- Outline the immediate management plan in the patient.
- Outline the subsequent management plan.

These tasks cover the domains as discussed next.

Core Clinical Skills Domains

Core clinical skills domains tested:

- Patient safety
- Communication with colleagues
- Application of knowledge.

Module Tested

The module tested in this station is Module 3 or 'Post-operative Care'.

EXAMINER'S INSTRUCTIONS AND STRUCTURED MARK SHEET

The examiner will mark the candidate on the basis of various tasks which are allotted to the candidate. Out of a total score of 20, the examiner would award a maximum of 20 marks, which are distributed between various candidate tasks as shown next. Each candidate task must be globally scored by the examiner.

Clinical Features Indicative of Shock in this Case

The patient may be in shock as evidenced by her hypotension and tachycardia. In addition, she may appear pale, sweaty and moist, and have cold and clammy extremities. The urine output is also reduced or absent in cases of shock. Other features which may be present include the following:

- Anxiety or agitation
- Confusion
- General weakness
- Rapid breathing.

Marking Scheme

0	1	2	3	4	5
Fail		Borderline		Pass	

Causes of her Shock

The likely causes for shock in this case include the following:

- *Haemorrhage (concealed or revealed)*: Haemorrhage can be concealed or revealed. In cases of revealed haemorrhage, the degree of shock would be proportional to the amount of blood lost. On the other hand, in concealed haemorrhage, no obvious bleeding is observed. Since in this case, no obvious bleeding was observed, the cause of haemorrhage is most likely to be concealed/or internal. Internal bleeding is evident from the vaginal examination, which is likely to reveal free fluid in the peritoneal cavity. This may be evident from the bogginess of the pouch of Douglas due to the accumulation of blood above the vaginal vault.
- *Drug reaction*: Drug reactions as a cause of the hypovolaemic shock will be evident from relationship between the time of onset of symptoms and the time of initiation of treatment. The most common drug involved is likely to be opiates, which are commonly used for providing post-operative analgesia. Other drugs may also cause shock; hence the medication which the patient is receiving must be reviewed thoroughly.
- *Infection*: Infections, especially Gram-negative bacteria, may cause septicaemia. The cases of Gram-negative septicaemia may be characterised by hypothermia and rashes.

- *Ureteric or bowel injury*: Although a rare cause of shock, injury to the bowel and/or ureters may present for the first time after surgery with features of shock.
- *Hypovolaemia due to inadequate fluid replacement*: Poor fluid replacement may also be a cause for hypovolaemic shock. This will be diagnosed by examining the deficit between fluid input and output in an input and output chart.

Marking Scheme

0	1	2	3	4	5
Fail		Borderline		Pass	

Outline of Immediate Management Plan

The immediate management steps involve the following:
- *Clinical examination*: A thorough physical examination should be undertaken to delineate various clinical features which could be suggestive of one of the causes of hypovolaemic shock (as discussed previously). The most important components of clinical examination in this case include an abdominal and pelvic examination, in which findings suggestive of free peritoneal fluid can be elicited.
- *Intravenous line*: Preferably with a large bore cannulae must be placed. In case there is already one cannula, another one with a large bore must be placed.
- *Intravenous fluids*: Fluid replacement should preferably be started with volume expanders. Adequate fluid replacement before or after surgical correction of any injury helps in reducing the risk of renal failure.[17]
- An urgent complete blood count along with the group and cross-match of at least 4 units of blood is required.
- The senior on call must be summoned because exploratory laparotomy may be required in this case.
- *The theatre staff and the anaesthetist must be called*: An exploratory laparotomy would be required in cases of suspected haemorrhage or bowel injury. Therefore, it is necessary to inform the anaesthetist and the theatre staff.
- Appropriate surgical staff belonging to other surgical specialities (e.g. bowel surgeons, urologists, etc.) may require to be called depending on the specific injury (e.g. injury to the bowel or the ureters). Surgical steps would be required based on the type of surgery performed depending on the type of injury incurred.

Marking Scheme

0	1	2	3	4	5
Fail		Borderline		Pass	

Outline of Subsequent Management Plan

- *Exploratory laparotomy*: An exploratory laparotomy will be required for suspected haemorrhage or bowel injury.
- *Rectification of the problem*: In case of injury to other organs, (e.g. bowel or ureter), appropriate specialities must be informed so that suitable surgical correction of the injury can be undertaken.

Marking Scheme

0	1	2	3	4	5
Fail		Borderline		Pass	

Total score: /20

DISCUSSION

Issues

One important issue involved in this station is to evaluate whether or not the candidate communicates with other medical professionals such as senior consultants, anaesthetists, surgeons, etc.

Another important issue which this station assesses is the manner in which the candidate applies clinical knowledge in form of management of hypovolemic shock in a post-operative patient.

Pitfalls

The common mistakes which the candidate can commit on such kind of station are failing to call for senior help or other medical colleagues such as the surgeon and anaesthetists. Another important mistake which can be committed on such kind of stations is just concentrating on the management of haemorrhage and ignoring other possible causes of hypovolemic shock as described previously.

Variations

There can be many variations in such kind of station where the candidate has to interact with different health care professionals such as paediatricians (e.g. in case of preterm labour or birth of a premature or growth restricted baby) or anaesthetists and surgeons (e.g. in case of various post-operative or intraoperative complications).

OSCE STATION 5: REFERRAL FROM A GP

Candidate's Instructions

A GP has referred a patient to the gynaecology clinic with the following letter. Read the letter below and then obtain the relevant history and discuss the management options with her. The examiner will provide you with additional information in case you require it.

Holly Tree Surgery
Wooden House Lane
Thorpes Beast Village
Walthome WN2 SU7
Dear Dr ......
Would you be kind enough to see this 28-year-old woman, Mrs Jodie Smith, who has history of infertility over the past 2 years? 1 year back, she was diagnosed as a case of mild endometriosis on laparoscopy. The endometriotic spots were observed on the uterosacral ligaments only and these lesions were coagulated using diathermy. The rest of the pelvis appeared normal. Jodie has been on a course of Provera for 9 months and is now asymptomatic. She has been recently diagnosed with human immunodeficiency virus (HIV) and has been put on triple antiviral therapy by the genitourinary medicine (GUM) physicians. Her CD4 count has improved significantly since she has been commenced on this therapy.
Thank you for your help.

Yours sincerely
Peter Pesh
DRCOG, MRCGP

The task is for 12 minutes (inclusive of 2 minutes of reading time). You have 10 minutes to counsel her about the situation. You shall be awarded marks for the following tasks:

Candidate's tasks:

- Take the relevant history from the patient
- Enlist the investigations which you would like to perform
- Results of some of investigations are described next. What management issues need to be considered in this case?
- What would you communicate with the GP in this case?

These tasks cover the domains as discussed next.

Core Clinical Skills Domains

Core clinical skills domains tested:

- Patient safety
- Communication with colleagues
- Information gathering
- Application of knowledge.

Module Tested

The module tested in this station is Module 10 or 'Subfertility'.

Role-player's Brief

You are a 28-year-old happily married woman, Mrs Jodie Smith, who works as a sales assistant. You have been with Brian, your husband, for 5 years and have regular intercourse, about 3–4 times a week. You have been trying to get pregnant since past 2 years.

- You underwent a laparoscopy 1 year back as an investigation for pain during intercourse. Your appendix was also removed at the age of 17 years. Besides these two surgeries, you have never undergone any other surgical procedure. The doctor diagnosed you to be a case of mild endometriosis and told you that the endometriotic lesions had been taken care of during surgery. Rest of your history is unremarkable.
- Your last cervical smear was done prior to your referral and the result was within normal limits.
- You used oral contraceptive pill in the past for 1 year after you got married.
- You are a non-smoker or non-alcoholic and you are not taking any kind of medication.
- Your partner is likewise fit and well and works as a bus driver. He smokes about 20 cigarettes per day and drinks a glass of wine with meals. He has not had any previous testicular problems and has never been a father of a child previously.
- You and your husband had planned pregnancy after 1–2 years of your marriage. However, now it has been 5 years of marriage and you have been trying for past 2 years. Presently, you are getting desperate to become pregnant because all your family and friends are expecting you to give them the 'good news'.
- The results of the various investigations performed in your case would suggest that there is a male factor involved. The candidate should explain the various options including the reproductive technologies as well as adoption to you.
- You feel your partner may get very upset at the thought that infertility is due to him.
- *Menstrual history*: Your last menstrual period occurred 3 weeks ago and you commenced your periods at the age of 12 years. Now, you have a regular 28-day cycle with bleeding for 5 days. You are not sure about the time when you ovulate, but offer this information only if the candidate asks about it.
- You had been an intravenous drug user (sharing needles) for 6 years but stopped last year.
- You have been recently diagnosed to be HIV positive and have been receiving three different drugs from the GUM clinic.

Prompt Questions

- Would it be ever possible for me to become pregnant in future?
- What are my options for becoming pregnant?
- How can my HIV positive status affect my pregnancy?

EXAMINER'S INSTRUCTIONS AND STRUCTURED MARK SHEET

The examiner will mark the candidate on the basis of various tasks which are allotted to the candidate. Out of a total score of 20, the examiner can award a maximum of 18 marks, which are distributed between various candidate tasks as shown next. The role-player can award a maximum of 2 marks to the candidate. Each candidate task must be globally scored by the examiner.

Examiner's Instructions

At this station, you should use the structured mark sheet to assess the candidate as he or she takes a history and discusses the management of the clinical problem with the role-player. You should only provide the additional information on examination if the candidate requests for it.

Taking the Relevant History

- Symptoms
- Duration
- Menstrual history
- Infertility or obstetric history
- *Past medical history*: Diagnosis of HIV infection and treatment
- *Past surgical history*: Laparoscopy for endometriosis
- *Social history*: She herself is non-alcoholic and non-smoker. On the other hand, husband is a smoker and occasionally drinks alcohol
- No history of testicular trauma and/or infection in the husband.

Marking Scheme

0	1	2	3	4
Fail	Borderline		Pass	

Investigations

- *Semen analysis*: For the evaluation of male factor infertility.
- *Mid-luteal phase progesterone levels*: For assessment of ovulation.
- *Hysterosalpingogram*: For evaluation of tubal patency.
- *Ultrasound examination*: For evaluation of uterine cavity and ovaries (for presence of any cysts, suggestive of polycystic ovaries).
- *High vaginal swab*: For detecting the presence of any abnormal micro-organisms.
- *Endocervical swab*: For evaluation of chlamydial infection.

Marking Scheme

0	1	2	3	4
Fail	Borderline		Pass	

Results of Various Investigations

For results of various investigations, see Tables 6.1 to 6.3.

Management Issues to be discussed with the Patient

- Results of various investigations in the woman are within normal limits.
- Abnormality with the total number of motile sperms and sperm concentration (points towards male factor infertility).

TABLE 6.1: Results of various investigations of Jodie Smith.

Investigations	Results
Day 21 progesterone level	75 IU/L
Hysterosalpingogram	• The uterus is normal anteverted and mobile. Both uterine tubes fill and the isthmus and ampullary portions appear normal. • There is free spill of contrast into the peritoneal cavity bilaterally with little retention of dye.
Pelvic ultrasound	• Normal anteverted uterus, with normal looking ovaries • No pelvic pathology seen and no evidence of polycystic ovary • Small amount of fluid in the Pouch of Douglas
HVS (high vaginal swab)	Presence of normal commensals
Endocervical swab	Negative for chlamydia

TABLE 6.2: Results of the semen analysis of Brian Smith (Jodie Smith's husband).

Collection	Masturbation
Days for abstinence	2 days
Time since production	90 minutes
Volume	2.8 mL
Viscosity	Normal
Motility	30%
Sperm concentration	0.6 million/mL
Abnormal form	50%
Non-sperm cell concentration	0.3 million/mL
Total motile sperm	0.5 million
Tray agglutination test	No antisperm antibody detected

TABLE 6.3: Results of the repeat semen analysis of Brian Smith (Jodie Smith's husband).

Collection	Masturbation
Days for abstinence	7 days
Time since production	45 minutes
Volume	3.8 mL
Viscosity	Normal
Motility	35%
Sperm concentration	0.9 million/mL
Abnormal form	55%
Non-sperm cell concentration	0.1 million/mL
Total motile sperm	2.4 million
Tray agglutination test	No antisperm antibody detected

- Do not discourage the role-player by saying that she may never get pregnant.
- Tell her that she may have difficulties in conceiving.
- Advise the husband to stop smoking; alcohol intake to be restricted.
- Advice about avoiding tight or restrictive underwear, avoiding hot water baths, and advising the use of multivitamins.
- Advise that intrauterine insemination (IUI) or donor insemination may not be very successful.
- Might require the use of assisted reproductive technologies [e.g. in vitro fertilisation (IVF)/intracytoplasmic sperm injection].
- According to the NICE (National Institute for Health and Care Excellence) guidelines, IVF should be available on the NHS and the couple would appear to be eligible.[18]
- Ask patient how far she wants to proceed, and mention that adoption may be an option.
- Since the patient is HIV positive, she requires counselling regarding both HIV and fertility treatment.
- She needs to be counselled regarding the chances of success.
- In case she conceives, steps need to be taken to prevent the vertical transmission of the HIV infection.

Marking Scheme

0	1	2	3	4	5	6
Fail		Borderline			Pass	

Communication with the GP

- Must mention about the various tests they have organised for the patient.
- The results of the various investigations need to be disclosed to the GP.
- Informs that they would be seeing the patient again within 3 months' time.
- Would keep the GP informed about the patient's progress.

Marking Scheme

0	1	2	3	4
Fail	Borderline		Pass	

Role-player's Score

The role-player can award a maximum of 2 marks to the candidate.

Marking Scheme

0	1	2
Role-player never wants to see candidate again	Role-player prepared to see candidate again	Role-player happy to see candidate again

Total score: /20

DISCUSSION

Issues

The consultants in the UK may often have to interact with the physicians in the primary care or the GPs. The patients who cannot be managed in the primary care are referred to the secondary care and subsequently to the tertiary care. In the MRCOG Part 3 examination, the candidates may be provided with a referral letter from the GP on the basis of which they have to treat the patient. The candidate would usually not be required to directly interact with the GP in the examination. The examiner may sometimes just ask the candidate if they would require more information from the GP or what they would like to communicate with the GP about the patient. However, in the real life scenario, there might be more direct communication with the GP through telephone calls, referral letters, etc.

Pitfalls

If at any point, the candidate feels that they require more information about the patient, they must ask the examiner. Failure to ask for such kind of information can be considered as a potential mistake.

This station is clearly a case of infertility due to a male factor. It is important that the candidate has an idea about the normal values of the common tests that are undertaken in the gynaecological outpatient clinic. In most cases the normal ranges will be given, but even so the candidate should have an idea about the normal range of the commonly requested tests (especially those associated with infertility). Failure to interpret the results of investigations in the absence of normal values can be considered as a potential mistake.

Variations

The patient could be referred to the secondary care for any ailment which could not be handled at the primary care. In the given scenario, the variation may be that the role-player may be the woman's husband and the candidate may have to discuss the result of reduced sperm count with him.

REFERENCES

1. National Confidential Enquiry into Patient Outcome and Death. Caring to the end? A review of the care of patients who died in hospital within four days of admission. NCEPOD; 2009.
2. Makeham M, Stromer S, Bridges-Webb C, et al. Patient safety events reported in general practice: a taxonomy. Qual Saf Health Care. 2008;17:53-7.
3. Hain P, Pichert JW, Hickson GB, et al. Using risk management files to identify and address causative factors associated with adverse events in paediatrics. Thera Clin Risk Manag. 2007;3:625-31.
4. Lingard L, Espin S, Whyte S, et al. Communication failures in the operating room: an observational classification of recurrent types and effects. Qual Saf Health Care. 2004;13:330-4.

5. Wiegmann DA, ElBardissi AW, Dearani JA, et al. Disruptions in surgical flow and their relationship to surgical errors: an exploratory investigation. Surgery. 2007;142:658-65.
6. Mazzocco K, Pettiti DB, Fong KT, et al. Surgical team behaviours and patient outcomes. Am J Surg. 2009;197:678-85.
7. Leonard M, Graham S, Bonacum D. The human factor: the critical importance of effective teamwork and communication in providing safe care. Qual Saf Health Care. 2004;13:85-90.
8. General Medical Council. Working with colleagues. [online] General Medical Council website. Available from http://www.gmc-uk.org/guidance/ethical_guidance/11811.asp [Accessed September 2017].
9. Breech presentation and delivery. In: Cunningham FG, Hauth JC, Leveno KJ, et al. (Eds). Williams Obstetrics, 24th edition. New York: McGraw-Hill Medical Publishing Division; 2014.
10. Royal College of Obstetrician and gynaecologists. (2015). Obtaining Valid Consent. Clinical Governance Advice No. 6. RCOG: London.
11. General Medical Council. (2008). Consent: patients and doctors making decisions together. [online] General Medical Council website. Available from www.gmc-uk.org/guidance [Accessed September 2017].
12. Yeomans ER. Operative vaginal delivery. Obstet Gynecol. 2010;115(3):645-53.
13. Feraud O. [Forceps: description, obstetric mechanics, indications and contra-indications]. J Gynecol Obstet Biol Reprod (Paris). 2008;37 Suppl 8:S202-9.
14. Dupuis O, Moreau R, Pham MT, et al. Assessment of forceps blade orientations during their placement using an instrumented childbirth simulator. BJOG. 2009;116(2):327-32; discussion 332-3.
15. Nikpoor P, Bain E. Analgesia for forceps delivery. Cochrane Database Syst Rev. 2013;9:CD008878.
16. William Whitaker. "William Whitaker's Words – Doctor". University of Notre Dame. [online] Available from http://www.archives.nd.edu/cgi-bin/wordz.pl?keyword=Doctor. [Accessed September 2017].
17. Shires GT. Management of hypovolemic shock. Bull N Y Acad Med. 1979;55(2):139-49.
18. National Institute of Clinical Excellence. (2013). Fertility problems: assessment and treatment. Clinical guideline [CG156]. NICE: London.

7

Information Gathering

INTRODUCTION

The most important skill involved in information gathering is history taking. This involves developing an understanding regarding what information is required and the method of obtaining that information. Taking an elaborate history is one of the most important skills which the candidates are taught at the medical school. They need to use this throughout their medical career as a fundamental method of gathering information. This approach eventually helps the doctor to create a differential diagnosis, thereby developing an appropriate plan for management.

In the scenario of an OSCE station, the proficient candidate will be expected to elicit information from the role-player or an actor, depicting the role of a simulated patient or trainee. Appropriate information is gathered using a combination of mainly open and some closed questions.

History taking is a core skill which is usually included during every examination. Though the candidates are expected to acquire a high-grade scoring for such kinds of stations, unexpectedly, the marks for these types of stations remain consistently low. It is important for the candidate to excel in the technique of taking a comprehensive history, not only of the presenting complaint but also all the relevant past histories, including medical history, surgical history, treatment history, and obstetric history. Medication history (including the history of taking alcohol, smoking, and recreational drug use) needs to be taken. Social history and family history may also be important especially in some scenarios. The candidate must follow a logical approach while taking history and not forget any of the components of history taking. Eliciting a detailed obstetric history is especially important in antenatal cases. In these cases, the doctor must elicit details regarding each of the previous pregnancies, carefully noting if there were any problems during the antenatal, intrapartum, and postpartum period, whether the labour was spontaneous or induced and whether the patient delivered normally or via a caesarean section. A record of baby's weight and sex must also be made. It is also important to make note of the pregnancies which ended in a failure (miscarriage, termination, intrauterine deaths or stillbirths). In case of miscarriages or termination, it is important to note the period of gestation when the event occurred, whether it was spontaneous or induced, whether or not any evacuations were performed, and occurrence of any post-operative complications.

While taking history, it is important for the candidate to notice the visual or facial cues given by the role-player. If you notice that the role-player continues to keep weeping, there is probably something which you have missed asking and needs to be addressed. The candidate must also not forget that the role-player may have been instructed to behave in a difficult or non-communicative manner in order to test your communication skills.

If a role-player is present at a particular station, it is important for the candidate not to interact with the examiner who would be merely present there as an observer and giving the candidate scoring on his marking sheet. If the candidates start interacting with the examiner, they are likely to break up the rapport that you have developed with the role-player. The candidate must not even approach the examiner if they have finished asking the questions and the consultation becomes silent. All the role-playing stations are designed in such a way that the examiner does not have any information for the candidate. They are just supposed to be present as the silent observer; all the necessary information on which the candidate would be scored will be on the instruction sheet. The marking scheme will be based on the issues, reflecting the information provided to the candidate.

While gathering information from the patient, the candidate must remember to follow the good practices as described by the General Medical Council.[1,2] These include the following:

- Introducing themselves
- Remaining professional at all times
- Staying in control of the consultation
- Confirming from the patient or role-player whether they have understood their questions or they have any questions which they want to ask.
- Effectively assess the patient's conditions, taking account of various factors such as clinical presentation, psychological, spiritual, social, and cultural factors.
- At all times the candidate must respect the patient's views and values.

At the end of the consultation, it is a good practice to summarise the information back to the role-player.

While preparing for such stations which require information gathering from the role-player, it is a good idea to practice with a friend or an exam buddy. Making a video recording while practicing on such stations and later carefully studying the video is a good idea.

OSCE STATION 1: GYNAECOLOGICAL HISTORY IN CASE OF UTERINE FIBROIDS

Candidate's Instructions

The patient you are about to see has been referred to your gynaecology outpatient clinic by her GP. A copy of the referral letter is given below. Read the letter and obtain appropriate history from the patient. You should discuss any relevant investigations and treatment options with the patient.

The Surgery
Barnston Road, Wirral
Merseyside CH61 1BW
Dear Gynaecologist
Please would you see Janice Hollingworth, a 42-year-old HIV-positive nulliparous woman presenting with menorrhagia. On general physical examination, she appears to be extremely pale. Abdominal examination has revealed a uterus with a size of 18 weeks. Her haemoglobin is found to be 9.0 g/dL. An ultrasound scan has revealed a large anterior fundal fibroid $12 \times 8 \times 6$ cm and a submucosal fibroid $7 \times 6 \times 4$ cm.
Thank you for your help.

Yours sincerely
Dr A Wilde (MRCGP)

The task is for 12 minutes (inclusive of 2 minutes of reading time). You have 10 minutes to counsel her about the situation. You shall be awarded marks for the following tasks:

Candidate's tasks:

- Take a relevant history from the patient
- What appropriate investigations you shall order in this case?
- What issues must you take into consideration while planning her treatment?
- Explain the management plan to the patient.

These tasks cover the domains as discussed next.

Core Clinical Skills Domains

Core clinical skills domains tested:

- Patient safety
- Communication with patients
- Communication with colleagues
- Information gathering
- Application of knowledge.

Module Tested

The module tested in this station is Module 9 or 'Gynaecological Problems.'

Role-player's Brief

- You are Janice Hollingworth, a 42-year-old HIV-positive nulliparous woman presenting with menorrhagia. You work as a music teacher in the primary school. You have a friendly and calm nature and are generally interested in finding out all about the benefits and risks of the treatment of your problem. You may, however, turn aggressive if someone is rude to you and demeans you, or if you are by and large dissatisfied with the doctor's attitude.
- You are worried that your bleeding may be related to the cancer of the womb because your sister died due to uterine cancer in her late 50s.
- Tell the doctor that you do not understand any medical terms. You must not interrupt the doctor unless you require some clarification and you let him or her lead the discussion.
- Your periods started when you were 12 years old, and since then had been regular until past 6 months. Your periods used to last for 4–5 days, and would come after every 28–30 days.
- However, over the last 6 months, you have noticed that your periods have largely become irregular. You experience bleeding between your periods and sometimes the bleeding suddenly starts when you are expected to be dry. You have to wear pads every day and remain generally worried.
- You do not experience any bleeding after sexual intercourse.
- Initially when your bleeding turned irregular, you met your GP who gave you some iron tablets but this did not cause any improvement.
- Your last cervical smear was done 2 years ago and that was normal.
- You have noticed over the past 3 months that you tend to become more tired and weak after performing normal activities. However, you have not experienced any shortness of breath, pain in the chest or palpitations.
- You have not been pregnant before as initially you and your husband wanted to enjoy a few years of your life after marriage all by yourself. Later you both decided that you do not want a baby. All this time you had been using contraception because you did not intend to get pregnant.
- You do not have any history of drug allergy.
- There is a family history of diabetes. Your mother suffers from type 2 diabetes, which is controlled with help of medication.
- There is also family history of cancer of the womb. Your sister was 59 years old when she was diagnosed with cancer of the womb at a late stage. A total abdominal hysterectomy and oophorectomy along with a debulking surgery was performed. She had died within 6 months of the diagnosis.
- You occasionally drink alcohol and do not smoke.

Prompt Questions

- Do I also have a cancer like my sister?
- What disorder do I have?
- Can my problem be treated?

EXAMINER'S INSTRUCTIONS AND STRUCTURED MARK SHEET

The examiner will mark the candidate on the basis of various tasks which are allotted to the candidate. Out of a total score of 20, the examiner can award a maximum of 18 marks, which are distributed between various candidate tasks as shown next. The role-player can award a maximum of 2 marks to the candidate. Each candidate task must be globally scored by the examiner.

History Taking

- Details of the patient's intermenstrual bleeding:
    - Date of her last menstrual period (LMP)
    - Amount of bleeding
    - Presence of associated symptoms (pain, weakness, etc.).
- Previous menstrual history including timing of her previous smear
- Previous obstetric history (including history of any fertility issues)
- Family history of any illness
- Past medical or surgical history
- Social history, including history of smoking, alcohol or abuse of recreational drugs
- History suggestive of anaemia
- History of post-coital bleeding.

Marking Scheme

0	1	2	3	4	5
Fail		Borderline		Pass	

Investigations

- Physical examination needs to be done if the patient's history is suggestive of any pathology.
    - Physical examination will help identify clinical anaemia
    - Identification of underlying causes of heavy menstrual bleeding such as thyroid masses and pelvic or abdominal masses
    - A mass in the pelvis, which is tender upon touching, is suggestive of endometriosis.
- Full blood count (FBC) requires to be done to exclude anaemia:
    - Blood group and save needs to be done if surgery is anticipated
    - Blood transfusion may be required if the patient is severely anaemic.
- Thyroid function test [measurement of free thyroxine (T4) levels and thyroid stimulating hormone (TSH) levels] must be undertaken in symptomatic patients.
- *Coagulation screen*: This may be performed if the patient had been complaining of heavy menstrual bleeding ever since menarche, and in case of a personal or family history suggestive of any coagulation defect.

> **BOX 7.1:** Indications for performing an ultrasound examination.
> - Uterus is palpable per abdomen
> - An adnexal mass is palpable on per abdominal or per vaginal examination
> - Failure of the medical treatment even in the absence of any palpable masses
> - Saline infusion sonography in the cases with suspected endometrial polyps

- *Pelvic ultrasound scan*: This would help in ruling out any ovarian or endometrial pathology. This investigation is especially important in this case because the uterus is palpable per abdomen. Ultrasound examination is also important in cases enlisted in Box 7.1. Another important reason for carrying out an ultrasound examination in this case is that the GP had tried medical treatment and this had failed.
- *Hysteroscopy*: This may be useful in cases where insufficient information is obtained on the ultrasound examination (e.g. the precise location or dimensions of a fibroid is unclear). Hysteroscopy is also important in cases where there is suspicion of malignancy (e.g. persistent intermittent bleeding or post-coital bleeding). In case of the suspicion of hyperplasia or malignancy, an endometrial biopsy should be performed at the time of hysteroscopy.
- *Blood glucose and glycosylated haemoglobin*: This is important in this case because the patient has a family history of diabetes.
- Cervical smear
- *Pipelle biopsy of endometrium ± hysteroscopy*: In this case, it is important to rule out carcinoma because the patient belongs to the perimenopausal age group and there is a history of intermenstrual bleeding.
- Assessment of possible therapeutic options, conservative, and surgical.

Marking Scheme

0	1	2	3	4
Fail		Borderline		Pass

Issues to be Considered while Planning her Treatment

- *Anaemia*: Heavy periods related to the presence of fibroids may be responsible for causing anaemia in this case. Also, surgical treatment can be undertaken only when the patient's haemoglobin levels have improved.
- *HIV infection*: General precautions must be taken to prevent the spread of infection to the staff. Also, in case surgical management is undertaken, steps must be taken to prevent the transmission of infection at the time of surgery.
  - Furthermore, the patient with HIV may be having an immuno-compromised status, which further increases risk of morbidity, e.g. infections, etc.
- *Parity*: Since the patient is nulliparous and not planning pregnancy in future, there is a low risk of transmission of the HIV infection to her children.

If the patient had been planning a pregnancy in future, there would have been a high risk of transmission of the HIV infection to her children. Since the patient is not desirous of future childbearing, there is no requirement of uterine conservative surgery.

- *Size of fibroids*: The fibroids in this case are very large and have caused the uterus to be palpable per abdomen. Since the fibroids are quite big in this case, there is a requirement for urgent removal because the large fibroids may cause pressure effects on the surrounding organs, e.g. ureter, rectum, etc.

Marking Scheme

0	1	2	3	4
Fail		Borderline		Pass

Management Options

- Since the patient's haemoglobin value is low, the most important aspect of her management requires provision of haematinic agents to correct her anaemia.
- The treatment of fibroids must be instituted on an emergency basis in view of the pressure symptoms caused by the large size of the fibroids.
- Irrespective of the treatment strategy, the GUM team must be involved in her care.
- The various treatment options which can be employed in this patient are described next.

Medical Treatment

- Medical treatment for fibroids comprises of medicines such as gonadotropin-releasing hormone (GnRH) agonists, danazol, (not recommended in the UK), etc. GnRH agonists help in downregulating the pituitary gland, thereby inducing amenorrhoea. Taking into account the patient's HIV status, anaemia, and the size of the fibroids, medical management is likely to serve as the best approach as well as the most cost-effective treatment strategy in this case.
- Another reason for the medical management to serve as the first line of management for this patient is as follows:
  - She is the perimenopausal age group and shall be approaching the menopause soon. Fibroids are known to naturally undergo a reduction in their size following menopause. Meanwhile, until the menopause is attained, use of GnRH agonists is likely to cause as much as 60% reduction in the size of fibroids and may serve as an acceptable option until the menopause sets it. This may also help in providing symptomatic relief and/or benefitting further surgery, in case it is considered. Since the woman belongs to perimenopausal age group, it may be possible to maintain her on this regimen, thereby avoiding surgery.

- The GnRH agonists also help in creating a state of amenorrhoea, thereby allowing her haemoglobin levels to rise and correction of her anaemic status.
- However, the patient may discontinue this treatment due to the presence of menopausal symptoms (especially osteopenia) associated with the long-term use of GnRh agonists. If this is the case, use of add-back therapy may prove to be a useful option. However, she should be warned against discontinuation of the GnRH therapy, because the fibroids are likely to regrow once the therapy is discontinued.
- Use of medical management is also associated with a minimal risk of HIV transmission to the staff.

Surgical Management

- In case of the failure of medical management, surgery would serve as the treatment of choice.
- The definitive surgery depends on the patient's requirement for fertility:
  - *Hysterectomy*: In case the patient is not desirous of future childbearing, hysterectomy is likely to serve as the surgery of choice. However, her anaemia needs to be corrected prior to this. This can be achieved through the prescription of GnRH agonists prior to the surgery to reduce the fibroid size as well as vascularity. Another advantage of hysterectomy is that it is associated with a reduced risk of disease transmission to the staff in comparison to myomectomy. This surgery would help in removing all the fibroids and avoiding the recurrence of anaemia.
  - *Myomectomy*: Myomectomy would serve as the operation of choice in case she had been desirous of future childbearing. However, myomectomy is likely to be associated with an increased risk of HIV transmission to the staff. Also, it may be associated with complications such as excessive haemorrhage and a requirement for eventually proceeding to hysterectomy. Besides, the remaining fibroids not removed by myomectomy have a tendency to regrow.

    If myomectomy needs to be undertaken in an HIV-positive patient, steps to be taken to minimise blood loss at the time of surgery are listed in Box 7.2.

BOX 7.2: Steps to be taken to minimise blood loss at the time of myomectomy.

Preoperative period:
- Use of gonadotropin-releasing hormone agonist or danazol for 3 months prior to the surgery (shrinkage of the fibroids as well as the reduction of vascularity, but results in an increased difficulty in shelving the fibroids and subsequent conversion to hysterectomy)

At the time of surgery:
- Use of Shirodkar's clamp or Bonney's myomectomy clamp (for temporary occlusion of the uterine arteries)
- Use of rubber tourniquet
- Injection of vasopressins (to reduce the blood loss)
- Transfixation of the uterine arteries

Interventional radiology: Uterine artery embolisation (UAE) does not serve as an option for women who are still planning to have a family.

- In the present case, UAE may not serve as an effective option due to the presence of large fibroids. The procedure, however, is associated with a minimal risk of transmission of the HIV infection to staff.
- Uterine artery embolisation requires technical expertise on the part of the surgeon. Long-term follow-up data regarding the efficacy of the procedure is yet not available. Also this technique is mainly available in tertiary centres where there is continuing research. Additionally, the procedure may be associated with its inherent complications, such as infection, persistent vaginal discharge, postembolisation syndrome—pain, nausea, vomiting, and fever (not involving hospitalisation), premature ovarian failure, haematoma, etc. Less commonly, the patient may have requirement for additional surgery following UAE.
- In this patient, UAE may be offered as the option of choice if medical options fail and the patient denies surgery.

Marking Scheme

0	1	2	3	4	5
Fail		Borderline		Pass	

Role-player's Score

The role-player can award a maximum of 2 marks to the candidate.

Marking Scheme

0	1	2
Role-player never wants to see candidate again	Role-player prepared to see candidate again	Role-player happy to see candidate again

Total score: /20

DISCUSSION

It is important to carefully take history of this patient because some important factors, which would be elicited at the time of history taking, need to be taken into consideration while planning her treatment. These factors include anaemia, her HIV status, parity, and the size of her fibroids. Her anaemia is probably related to the heavy periods secondary to her fibroids. Treatment of menorrhagia due to fibroids is likely to correct her anaemia. She needs to be prescribed some oral haematinics for correction of her anaemia. Prescription of GnRH agonists is like to reduce the size as well as the vascularity of the fibroids, thereby reducing the blood loss.[3] However, medical management with GnRH analogues results in temporary effects, i.e. the fibroids have a tendency to regrow. Therefore, it is best to administer GnRH agonists prior to surgery to help reduce the size of the fibroids.

Her HIV status also poses an important problem for the clinician. She presents a significant risk of transmission of HIV infection to the staff especially if she is undergoing myomectomy due to a high risk of haemorrhage associated with this surgery. Moreover, she is likely to be immunocompromised. She would be at an increased risk of acquired infections, especially in hospital following invasive management. She is nulliparous and is not desirous of future childbearing. Therefore, there is no need to conserve her uterus while planning her treatment. The location, size, and number of her fibroids would help in deciding the treatment which would be best suitable for her.[4]

Issues

Taking a gynaecological history is a core skill for an MRCOG candidate. This is a skill which the doctors practice every day and they need to be very good at it. Despite of this, sometimes candidates score very badly on history-taking stations. The candidates need to remember that they would be tested on their history taking and communication skills. Therefore, while preparing for part 3 examination, they particularly need to practice history taking and communication skills while rehearsing with their exam buddy. If they have practiced well in advance, they are unlikely to give up under the stress of the examinations.

In these stations the role-player may have been briefed to be difficult and may try to lead the candidate up to the wrong path. The candidate can deal with this problem through adoption of good communication and history taking skills.

Pitfalls

The most important mistake which the candidate can commit in this case is listing the various treatment options, without critically appraising them in context to the patient's history. This may result due to the candidate's poor history taking skills, which is likely to result in a potential failure. Forgetting to enquire about family history, social history, and history of alcohol and illicit drug use can be considered as an important mistake.

Since in this station, the candidates have not been provided with the results of various investigations, they need to propose the treatment options depending on the probable results of the investigation. The candidate must also clearly think about getting this kind of information across to the patient in a manner they can understand. It may be sometimes helpful to explain the patient with the help of diagrams.

Failure to justify the actions you shall take in this patient can also be considered as an important mistake.

Variations

History-taking stations could be pertaining to several gynaecological problems (including menstrual disorders, endocrine disorders, disorders of puberty, congenital anomalies, menopause, management of gynaecological emergencies, etc.). The candidate needs to be well versed with all these situations.

OSCE STATION 2: OBSTETRIC HISTORY

Candidate's Instructions

The patient you are about to see is Mrs Susan Tyler, 29 years old, who has been referred to your antenatal clinic by her GP. A copy of the referral letter is given below.

The Surgery
High Street, Sheffield, S1 2GE
Dear Doctor,
Re: Mrs Susan Tyler, 29 years old
Would you please book Mrs Susan Tyler for antenatal care? She is 29 years old and 26 weeks pregnant. This is her second pregnancy. I have enclosed some of the investigation results.
Yours sincerely
Dr Beattie (MRCGP)

Investigations (Susan Tyler, 29 years old)
- Blood group: B, Rh-negative
- FBC: Normal
- VDRL: Negative
- Rubella: Immune
- Mid-stream urine (MSU): No growth
- Ultrasound examination (done in the first trimester) shows single live intrauterine pregnancy consistent with 11 weeks gestation; no other abnormalities detected.

The task is for 12 minutes (inclusive of 2 minutes of reading time). You have 10 minutes to read the mentioned letter from the GP and obtain a relevant history from the patient. The GP's examination of the patient should be taken to be unremarkable. You shall be awarded marks for the following tasks:

Candidate's tasks:
- Obtain an obstetric history and risk factors
- Discuss relevant and appropriate investigations which need to be done in this case
- Outline the adverse effects of these on her pregnancy
- Discuss the appropriate steps of management.

These tasks cover the domains as discussed next.

Core Clinical Skills Domains

Core clinical skills domains tested:
- Patient safety
- Communication with patients
- Communication with colleagues
- Information gathering
- Application of knowledge.

Module Tested

The module tested in this station is Module 4 or 'Antenatal Care'.

Role-player's Brief

- You are Susan Tyler, a 29-year-old woman, who works in the sex industry. You have been happily married since last 5 years and live with your husband. You are pregnant for the second time and your first child is 5 years old girl. In your second pregnancy, you have reached 26 weeks' gestation. Your expected date of delivery (EDD) is 14 weeks later.
- You first started having your periods when you were 13 years old. Since then your periods have been regular and occur after every 28 days with the bleeding lasting for 4–5 days. You had been using intrauterine contraceptive device for contraception, but this pregnancy was due to contraception failure.
- Though you are not sure about the date of your LMP, you are 26 weeks of gestation today as per the calculation based on the ultrasound scan done at 11 weeks of gestation.
- This is your second pregnancy and so you are confident about the situation. You are assured that you shall be able to well deal with it. You cannot stand people who exert authority over you. You visualise the doctor as an authority figure and therefore you would not be easy to handle during the interview.
- Last cervical smear was done about 5 years ago.
- You smoke nearly 20 cigarettes a day.
- You occasionally consume alcohol (approximately 1 unit per week).
- You occasionally also smoke marijuana and cocaine, but there is no history of intravenous drug usage.
- *Allergies*: There is no significant history of allergies.
- *Drugs taken*: You have been taking folic acid during entire period of gestation until now.
- *Surgical history*: There is no significant history of surgery in the past.
- *Medical history*: You suffered from congenital dislocation of the hip as a baby. As a result you had successive recurring hip problems in the childhood.

Prompt Questions

- Is my pregnancy at high risk?
- Will my baby be malformed?

EXAMINER'S INSTRUCTIONS AND STRUCTURED MARK SHEET

The examiner will mark the candidate on the basis of various tasks which are allotted to the candidate. Out of a total score of 20, the examiner can award a maximum of 18 marks, which are distributed between various candidate tasks as shown next. The role-player can award a maximum of 2 marks to the candidate. Each candidate task must be globally scored by the examiner. Familiarise yourself with the candidate's instructions and the role-player's brief.

Candidates should discuss with the patient any relevant investigations they feel are appropriate. Investigations that need to be considered by the candidate in view of the patient's occupation are:

- Hepatitis B and C screen
- HIV test
- Cervical smear
- High vaginal swab (HVS) and *Chlamydia* swabs.

Obstetric History

- Basic obstetric history including date of LMP, EDD, duration of marriage, any previous children, miscarriages, etc.
- Is the pregnancy a planned one and how is it progressing till date?
- Any previous medical, surgical or family history of significance.
- Her occupation and her social history including history of smoking, alcohol consumption, recreational drug use, domestic violence, etc.

Risk Factors

- Convey the fact that she may be at risk of HIV and substance abuse (due to her occupation).
- The importance of attending for routine antenatal check-ups must be emphasised to her.
- She is Rh negative. Therefore, she would require appropriate antibody checks-ups and administration of anti-D immune globulins during the pregnancy.
- Patient is at a high risk of developing sexually transmitted diseases.
- Risks related to smoking, and use of recreational drugs on the pregnancy need to be explained to her.

Marking Scheme

0	1	2	3	4	5	6
Fail		Borderline		Pass		

Relevant Investigations

- Routine investigations done, including FBC, group, rubella, and syphilis
- HIV screening
- Cervical cytology
- *Chlamydia* testing and HVS
- Hepatitis B and C screen
- A detailed anomaly scan.

Marking Scheme

0	1	2	3	4
Fail		Borderline		Pass

TABLE 7.1: Adverse effects for both mother and the baby.

Maternal	Foetal

Pregnancy-related complications:
• Miscarriages
• Foetal growth restriction
• Placental abruption
• Intrauterine death or hypoxia
• Preterm labour
Medical complications:
• Chronic lung disease
• Venous thromboembolism
• Long-term consequences include lung cancer and arterial disease, heart failure, heart attacks, chronic malnutrition and chronic obstructive airway disease, maternal death, etc.
	Foetal complications:
	• Miscarriage
	• Preterm labour
	• Intrauterine foetal death
	• Placental abruption
	• Intrauterine hypoxia
	• Prolonged pregnancy
	Newborn/infant:
	• Neonatal death:
	  – Cot death
	  – Early neonatal death
	• Long-term neurodevelopmental disability
	• Poorer intellect
	• Reduced intelligence
	• Short attention span and hyperactivity
	• Increased neonatal morbidity and mortality
	• Polycythaemia, which may be complicated by neonatal venous thrombosis and associated mortality

Adverse Effects of the Risk Factors on her Pregnancy

• Consequences of smoking and other drugs of abuse need to be explained to her.
• Smoking produces nicotine and carboxyhaemoglobin. These cross the placenta and circulate within the foetus, resulting in the adverse effects for both mother and the baby (Table 7.1).[5-8]

Marking Scheme

0	1	2	3	4
Fail		Borderline		Pass

Steps for Management

• Besides the routine antenatal care, the main step of managing this patient involves persuading her to give up smoking during pregnancy.
• The first step in encouraging this woman to give up smoking is to educate her regarding the harmful outcomes of smoking on her baby as well as on herself.
• The next step involves offering support and alternative means for giving up smoking to the patient. She may also be advised to use nicotine patches and gum, which may act as a substitute whenever she experiences craving for a cigarette.
• The doctor also needs to counsel the patient's partner or family members regarding the adverse effect of smoking. They must be emphasised about their role in supporting her. Providing information pertaining to the

several maternal and neonatal side effects (especially sudden infant death syndrome or cot death) associated with smoking is likely to help alleviate this problem.

- The patient must be informed that the though smoking does not result in a specific congenital anomaly this does not imply that the baby would be born healthy. Sometimes smoking may result in less obvious consequences, which may manifest only later in life.
- Support and counselling of such patients should be preferably provided by experts (e.g. support groups, midwives, social workers, etc.) who are specifically devoted towards supporting and counselling such patients.

Marking Scheme

0	1	2	3	4
Fail		Borderline		Pass

Role-player's Score

The role-player can award a maximum of 2 marks to the candidate.

Marking Scheme

0	1	2
Role-player never wants to see candidate again	Role-player prepared to see candidate again	Role-player happy to see candidate again

Total score: /20

DISCUSSION

Issues

This station tests the ability of the candidate to take a basic obstetric history and to establish the risks for this patient and her pregnancy. Capability of taking a basic obstetric history is a core skill which the candidate attempting the part 3 examination is expected to know. Once the correct questions have been asked, any relevant investigations and appropriate management should ensue. A good candidate would be able to effectively elicit the various risk factors which may ensue in this seemingly normal pregnancy at the time of taking history. This must be followed by instituting relevant investigations and appropriate management. Some of the risk factors which need to be elicited in this case include: Rh-negative status, antibody screen and immunization with anti-D immune globulins; high risk of sexually transmitted diseases; risk of an abnormal smear; risk associated with smoking, and the possibility of drug abuse. The candidate must be aware about the routine screening blood tests that are done in the UK.

In this case, the GP's examination is taken to be normal and therefore, the candidate is not expected to interact with the examiner. The examiner's role would be just to mark the candidate according to the prescribed mark sheet.

The role-player has been given a scenario and will answer questions when asked. Since this is a straightforward station, the role-player may have been instructed to make it difficult for the candidate. She would have been briefed regarding how much help she can provide to the candidates. She might have been provided with the list of specific questions to ask candidates. A particular role-player may be instructed to behave as a 'nightmare patient' and the examiner may be marking the candidate on how they deal with that particular patient.

The various recommendations by NICE (National Institute for Health and Care Excellence) guidelines for care of pregnant women who smoke are tabulated in Table 7.2. According to the first recommendation by the NICE guidelines, midwives must identify the pregnant women who smoke and refer them to National Health Services (NHS) Stop Smoking Services.[9] The Stop Smoking Service team offers one-to-one appointments to the woman and also helps suggest ways to help her cope up with her cravings and withdrawal symptoms, which may occur once she stops smoking. The length of time for which the woman may require support would vary for each woman and may depend on her circumstances. Typically, a 12-week programme is likely to be useful to most women through their initial period. The referral pathway from maternity services to NHS Stop Smoking Services is illustrated in Flow chart 7.1.[9]

Pitfalls

The major difficulty the candidates may face with such types of station is that, in the UK, a midwife mostly takes full obstetric history, so the candidate may

TABLE 7.2: Recommendations by NICE guidelines.[9]

Recommendations	Specifications
Recommendation 1	Action for midwives—identifying pregnant women who smoke and referring them to NHS Stop Smoking Services
Recommendation 2	Action for others in the public, community, and voluntary sectors (GPs, practice nurses, health visitors, family nurses, obstetricians, paediatricians, sonographers and other members of the maternity team other than the midwives)—identifying pregnant women who smoke and referring them to NHS Stop Smoking Services
Recommendation 3	Stop Smoking Services—contacting referrals (NHS Stop Smoking Services specialist advisers should contact all referrals on telephone)
Recommendation 4	Stop Smoking Services—initial and ongoing support to be provided by the NHS Stop Smoking Services specialist advisers. This involves offering women the following interventions to help them quit smoking: cognitive behaviour therapy, motivational interviewing and structured self-help, and support from NHS Stop Smoking Services
Recommendation 5	Use of NRT and other pharmacological support
Recommendation 6	NHS Stop Smoking Services—meeting the needs of disadvantaged pregnant women who smoke
Recommendation 7	Meeting the needs of partners and others in the household who smoke
Recommendation 8	Training to deliver interventions

(GPs: general practitioners; NHS: National Health Service; NRT: nicotine replacement therapy)

Flow chart 7.1: The referral pathway from maternity services to National Health Service Stop Smoking Services.

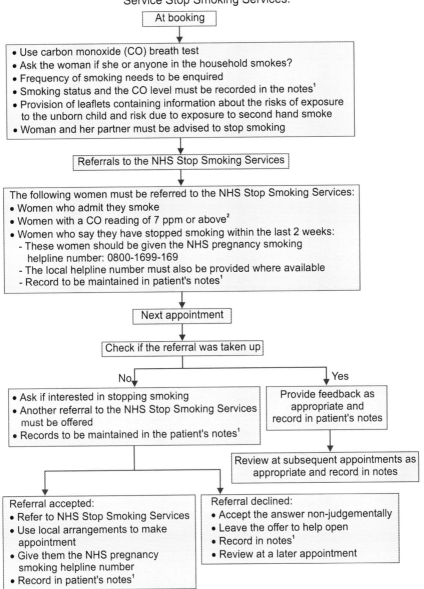

At booking

- Use carbon monoxide (CO) breath test
- Ask the woman if she or anyone in the household smokes?
- Frequency of smoking needs to be enquired
- Smoking status and the CO level must be recorded in the notes[1]
- Provision of leaflets containing information about the risks of exposure to the unborn child and risk due to exposure to second hand smoke
- Woman and her partner must be advised to stop smoking

Referrals to the NHS Stop Smoking Services

The following women must be referred to the NHS Stop Smoking Services:
- Women who admit they smoke
- Women with a CO reading of 7 ppm or above[2]
- Women who say they have stopped smoking within the last 2 weeks:
  - These women should be given the NHS pregnancy smoking helpline number: 0800-1699-169
  - The local helpline number must also be provided where available
  - Record to be maintained in patient's notes[1]

Next appointment

Check if the referral was taken up

No
- Ask if interested in stopping smoking
- Another referral to the NHS Stop Smoking Services must be offered
- Records to be maintained in the patient's notes[1]

Yes
Provide feedback as appropriate and record in patient's notes

Review at subsequent appointments as appropriate and record in notes

Referral accepted:
- Refer to NHS Stop Smoking Services
- Use local arrangements to make appointment
- Give them the NHS pregnancy smoking helpline number
- Record in patient's notes[1]

Referral declined:
- Accept the answer non-judgementally
- Leave the offer to help open
- Record in notes[1]
- Review at a later appointment

Notes: 1. Preferably the patient's hand held records; 2. Lower level (e.g. 3 ppm) may apply for light or infrequent smokers.

not have been routinely exposed to history taking during their clinical training. It is therefore important for the candidate to practice such types of OSCE stations while preparing for the part 3 examination. With any obstetric history it is important to elicit key points such as the patient's occupation, whether this was a planned pregnancy or not, menstrual history, smear history, etc.

Since antenatal care involves routine screening, it is important to appreciate this fact at the time of taking a history. Not taking the patient's social history including, including tobacco, alcohol consumption, and use of recreational drugs can be considered as an important pitfall.

With any pregnancy (whether low risk or high risk), the candidate would be required to formulate a plan of action (including the investigations required) and a management decision.

Another important thing which needs to be remembered by the candidates during such role-player stations is to avoid the use of medical jargon, especially abbreviations. The actors which have been selected as role-players are not medical personnel and they may not understand the medical terms. Therefore, use of medical terminology by the candidate while explaining to the role-player can be considered as an important mistake.

Variations

The candidate's history taking skill can not only be tested in a normal patient but a wide variety of scenarios including those having some obstetric complication such as twin gestation, Rh-negative pregnancy, malpresentation, previous history of caesarean delivery, antepartum haemorrhage, foetal growth restriction, etc. or presence of medical complications such as pre-eclampsia, gestational diabetes, heart disease, haematological disorders, etc.

OSCE STATION 3: ANTENATAL HISTORY

Candidate's Instructions

The patient you are about to see is Mrs Nazia Khan, a 30-year-old Pakistani woman. She has been referred to your antenatal clinic by her GP. A copy of the referral letter is given below.

Surgery,
Station Road,
London SW13 0LW, UK
Dear Doctor,
Re: Mrs Nazia Khan
Please see and book this 30-year-old Pakistani woman for antenatal care.
She has been in the UK for past 12 years and speaks limited English. She is gravida 6, para 3 and two miscarriages. She has had three full-term normal deliveries over the past 10 years; her youngest child is 3 year old. She is currently 11 weeks pregnant, which has been confirmed by a first trimester ultrasound scan.
Her history is otherwise unremarkable. She is keen to visit Pakistan this week because her brother has met with a near fatal accident. She would like your advice regarding air travel.

Yours sincerely
Dr Lawrence (MRCGP)

The task is for 12 minutes (inclusive of 2 minutes of reading time). You have 10 minutes to counsel her about the situation. You shall be awarded marks for the following tasks:

> **Candidate's tasks:**
> - Obtain a relevant obstetric history from the patient
> - Establish a plan of management for this pregnancy
> - Address any patient concerns.

The general examination of this patient is normal for her gestation. This station tests the candidate's skill for taking an obstetric history and their communication skills with regard to the management.

These tasks cover the domains as discussed next.

Core Clinical Skills Domains

> **Core clinical skills domains tested:**
> - Patient safety
> - Communication with patients
> - Communication with colleagues
> - Information gathering
> - Application of knowledge.

Module Tested

The module tested in this station is Module 4 or 'Antenatal Care'.

Role-player's Brief

- You are Nazia Khan, a 30-year-old Pakistani woman, who moved into the UK with your husband after marriage at the age of 18 years.
- Despite of staying in the UK since past 12 years, your English is limited and you may require an interpreter. You occasionally work as a part time helper in a hospice charity shop adjacent to your house.
- You are gravida 6, para 3 and had two miscarriages in the past. You have had three full-term normal deliveries over the past 10 years and your youngest child is 3 years old boy. All your deliveries took place in the UK in the hospital.
- You had your first child, a baby girl, when you were 20 years old. The baby delivered normally at term via vaginal route. You had no complications during the antenatal, intrapartum or the postpartum period.
- When you were aged 25 years, you delivered another baby girl at 37 weeks of gestation. Though the antepartum period had been largely normal, you remember having lot of pain and bleeding, once your waters broke while you were at home. You were immediately taken to the hospital. However, you delivered quickly, once in the hospital. The baby did not cry immediately after birth and was kept in the neonatal nursery for 24 hours.
- Three years ago you delivered another child, this time a baby boy. You, however, did not receive regular antenatal care during this pregnancy because there were a lot of family issues and you had been under a lot of stress. You saw a doctor at 28 weeks of gestation because you developed severe headache. You were referred to the hospital where you were

diagnosed as a case of hypertension. You were admitted in the hospital for a week and started on anti-hypertensive medicines, following which your blood pressure came under control. All this while, the doctor told you that your child had been slightly growth restricted. You delivered a male infant weighing 2.3 kg at 38 weeks of gestation. The baby was active after birth and was handed over to you immediately.

- All these deliveries were planned ones and now you have three children, the eldest being a 10-year-old girl, second is a 5-year-old girl, and the youngest one is 3-year-old boy.
- You have had two miscarriages, one 6 months after your marriage and another one a year back. Both the miscarriages occurred spontaneously at 8–10 weeks of gestation. You did not visit the doctor after both these miscarriages and no surgical intervention was done following either of these miscarriages as you felt that you had delivered the gestational sac completely.
- Your periods first started when you were 10 years old. Your periods are regular, and you have been bleeding for 4–5 days every 28 days. You have never had a cervical smear test done in the past.
- You do not smoke cigarettes and drink only occasionally.
- There is no medical history of note. You are unaware of your blood group.
- There is no significant family history.
- Your present pregnancy is a planned one. You had some bleeding in early pregnancy. As a result an ultrasound examination was performed. You are sure of your period of gestation due to the report of ultrasound.
- There have been no other problems so far in this pregnancy.
- You are keen to visit Pakistan this week because your brother has met with a near fatal accident you would like the doctor's advice regarding air travel.

Prompt Questions

- Will travelling to Pakistan affect my pregnancy in any way?
- Do I need to take any extra precautions?

EXAMINER'S INSTRUCTIONS AND STRUCTURED MARK SHEET

The examiner will mark the candidate on the basis of various tasks which are allotted to the candidate. Out of a total score of 20, the examiner can award a maximum of 18 marks, which are distributed between various candidate tasks as shown next. The role-player can award a maximum of 2 marks to the candidate. Each candidate task must be globally scored by the examiner.

History Taking

- General obstetric history:
  - Planned or unplanned pregnancy?
  - Does she have a good family support?
- Date of her LMP and expected due date of delivery.
- A detailed obstetric history.

- Past medical and surgical history.
- Social history including the history of smoking, alcohol, and substance abuse.
- Treatment history: Past or present history of treatment with some drug.
- Smear history: Since she has never had a cervical smear test done in the past, the patient may require an opportunistic smear (during the time of antenatal check-up).

Obstetric History

- *History of first pregnancy*: Normal vaginal delivery. Antepartum, intra-partum, and postpartum periods were uneventful.
- Normal foetal weight in first pregnancy.
- Second pregnancy was suggestive of the history of placental abruption.
- History of pre-eclampsia in the third pregnancy. The foetus was growth restricted and born with a low body weight. The baby, however, was born alert with an APGAR score of 8.

Marking Scheme

0	1	2	3	4	5	6
Fail		Borderline		Pass		

Management During Pregnancy

- Checking the patient's blood group and antibody status:
  - In case of Rh negative pregnancy, the patient may require tertiary referral depending upon the antibody levels in the blood.
- Checking the patient's blood pressure and urine sample for the presence of proteins.
- Monitoring the foetal growth.
- She should be booked up for routine antenatal check-ups.
- Supplementation with folic acid should be begun.
- Routine antenatal blood investigations (e.g. haemoglobin levels, etc.).
- All antenatal screening, including screening for haemoglobinopathies, the foetal anomaly scan, screening for Down's syndrome, screening for infectious diseases (HIV, hepatitis B and syphilis), etc.

Marking Scheme

0	1	2	3	4	5	6
Fail		Borderline		Pass		

Addressing the Patient on Air Travel during Pregnancy[10]

- Air travel during pregnancy usually does not present a risk to a healthy pregnant woman.

- International travel usually does not present with any problem until 32–35 weeks of gestation. The patient should be, however, advised to carry her antenatal notes along with the EDD and appropriate insurance.
- Presently, there is no evidence to suggest that air flight would cause complications such as miscarriage, early labour or premature rupture of membranes. She is at the risk of having a miscarriage (1 in 5) in the first 3 months of pregnancy, whether or not she flies.
- The patient should be advised to fasten the seat belt at the pelvic level or below her baby bump.
- While in the flight, she should be advised to walk every 30 minutes.
- While sitting in the plane, the woman must be asked to frequently flex and extend her ankles.
- To overcome the dehydrating effect of low humidity in the aircraft, she must be advised to substantially consume fluids.
- It is important to exclude any potential underlying medical problems before giving any further advice about travelling.
- Pregnant women or those in the postpartum period (6 weeks after pregnancy) are at a higher risk of developing a deep vein thrombosis (DVT) in comparison to the women who are not pregnant.
  To minimise the risk of a DVT on a medium or a long-haul flight (over 4 hours), the woman should be asked to observe the following precautions:
  - Wearing loose clothing and comfortable shoes
  - Trying to get an aisle seat, which provides more space in comparison to the other seats
  - Taking regular walks around the plane
  - Doing exercises of the ankles and feet while sitting on their seats every 30 minutes
  - Cutting down on drinks that contain alcohol or caffeine (coffee and fizzy drinks)
  - Wearing graduated elastic compression stockings.

Marking Scheme

0	1	2	3	4	5	6
Fail		Borderline		Pass		

Role-player's Score

The role-player can award a maximum of 2 marks to the candidate.

Marking Scheme

0	1	2
Role-player never wants to see candidate again	Role-player prepared to see candidate again	Role-player happy to see candidate again

Total score: /20

> **BOX 7.3:** The questions to be asked from the role-player.
> - The reason why the woman wants to fly at this particular time?
> - Is her flight necessary?
> - How long would be her flight?
> - How many weeks pregnant will she be when she travels and when shall she return?
> - Does she have any underlying medical problems?
> - What are the medical facilities available at the flight destination in case there is an unexpected complication with her pregnancy?
> - Has she got all the relevant immunisations and/or medication for the country she is travelling to?
> - Has she checked up with the airlines and travel insurance policies regarding whether the pregnancy and/or care for her newborn baby would be covered in case she gives birth unexpectedly?

DISCUSSION

Issues

This station again tests the candidate's history taking and counselling skills. The candidate is required to counsel the role-player about the risks which may be associated with air travel during pregnancy. Besides this, it is also important to take a detailed obstetric history to elicit factors in previous pregnancy which could affect the management decisions in the present pregnancy.

She must be explained about her options along with the pros and cons of each option. She should also be counselled about the support she can get to help her reach the correct decision. She must be advised that the safest time to fly is before 37 weeks, in case of a singleton pregnancy and before 32 weeks, in case she is carrying an uncomplicated twin pregnancy. The questions listed in Box 7.3 may also help the candidates in making their decision.

Pitfalls

Just concentrating on taking the patient's history and not addressing her concerns can be considered as a potential mistake in such kinds of stations.

Variations

As previously explained, there can be numerous variations involving several antenatal scenarios for such kind of stations. Also, in the similar station, variation can be introduced by changing the role-player's period of gestation.

OSCE STATION 4: SECONDARY AMENORRHOEA

Candidate's Instructions

Mrs Linda Lansbridge is a 28-year-old woman and has been referred with a history of secondary amenorrhoea since past 6 months by her GP. A copy of the referral letter is given below.

GP practice
Middlewich Road, Sandbach, Cheshire
CW11 1EQ
Dear Doctor,
Re: Mrs Linda Lansbridge, 28 years old
I request you to see Mrs Linda Lansbridge, a 28-year-old patient with a history of secondary amenorrhoea since past 6 months. She first experienced her periods at the age of 14 years. Her periods were regular and remained so until last 6 months, since when she has not been experiencing her periods. She and her husband are keen to start their family and have been trying since past 1 year. She is worried that she may not be able to conceive at all because she has stopped having her periods.

I have enclosed the results of some hormonal blood tests which I had ordered for her.

Yours sincerely
Dr Brett Mckinley (MRCGP)

Investigations (Mrs Linda Lansbridge, 28 years old)
- Follicle-stimulating hormone levels raised
- Progestogen challenge test is negative
- Prolactin levels: Within normal limits
- Thyroid function test: Within normal limits
- Pregnancy test is negative.

The task is for 12 minutes (inclusive of 2 minutes of reading time). You have 10 minutes to counsel her about the situation. You shall be awarded marks for the following tasks:

Candidate's tasks:
- Take relevant history from this patient
- What is likely differential diagnosis in this case on the basis of history and results of the investigations?
- Devise an appropriate management plan.

These tasks cover the domains as discussed next.

Core Clinical Skills Domains

Core clinical skills domains tested:
- Patient safety
- Communication with patients
- Communication with colleagues
- Information gathering
- Application of knowledge.

Module Tested

The module tested in this station is Module 9 or 'Gynaecological Problems'.

Role-player's Brief

- You are Mrs Linda Lansbridge, a 28-year-old woman with a history of absence of periods since past 6 months. You were referred by your GP.

- You are pursuing your PhD. You know you had been under stress as you are writing up your PhD thesis. Initially you thought that the absence of periods was related to your stressful lifestyle.
- Your periods first started when you were 14 years old. Your periods were regular and remained so until last 6 months, since when you have not been experiencing your periods.
- You have lately experienced some hot flushes and have also noticed some vaginal dryness with intercourse recently. Your periods have also stopped coming since past 6 months. Now you have really become worried because you and your husband had been planning a family.
- You went to see your GP 8 weeks ago about this problem and you had some hormonal blood tests taken. These blood tests have been repeated with no change in their values. You have been referred by your GP to discuss the consequences of the situation.
- You got married at the age of 24 years and had been using contraception until last year. Now you and your husband are keen to start their family and have been trying since past 1 year. You are worried that you may not be able to conceive at all because you have stopped having your periods.
- When you were 18 years old, you developed cough, trouble breathing, and chest pain. After having treated you for about 5–6 months for your nonspecific symptoms, the GP eventually referred you for a chest X-ray, which showed extensive shadowing and you were diagnosed as a case of Hodgkin's lymphoma. You underwent intensive treatment with several cycles of chemotherapy. Now you are clear of the disease.
- You have never been pregnant before.
- You had your appendix removed at the age of 6 years. Besides this there is no previous history of any surgery.
- Your mother underwent a total abdominal hysterectomy and removal of her ovaries for severe endometriosis when she was 42 years old. She was then started on hormone replacement therapy (HRT).
- You do not take any medication, and there is no history of any allergies.
- You do not smoke cigarettes nor do you consume alcohol.
- Your last cervical smear test was taken 2 years back and was found to be normal.
- Your grandmother developed pulmonary embolism after surgery for hip fracture at the age of 92 years. She survived for 15 days after surgery.
- You have never been pregnant in the past.
- There is no history of any milky discharge from breasts, history of weight gain or weight loss, acne, hair growth or deepening of voice.

Prompt Questions

- I want to know about my diagnosis.
- I am very concerned about my fertility.
- What are my chances of conceiving in future?

EXAMINER'S INSTRUCTIONS AND STRUCTURED MARK SHEET

The examiner will mark the candidate on the basis of various tasks which are allotted to the candidate. Out of a total score of 20, the examiner can award a maximum of 18 marks, which are distributed between various candidate tasks as shown next. The role-player can award a maximum of 2 marks to the candidate. Each candidate task must be globally scored by the examiner.

Taking Relevant History

- Age
- Menstrual history including the age of attaining menarche
- Obstetric history
- Current medication
- Weight loss and BMI
- Family history
- Current occupation
- Exercise levels
- Cervical smear test
- Fertility issues: How long she has been trying for a family, frequency of intercourse
- Previous history of medical problems
- Smoking and alcohol history
- *History of weight loss*: Stress-induced, exercise, and anorexia
- *History of hyperprolactinaemia*: Inappropriate galactorrhoea and headaches
- History of intake of drugs, especially steroids, anti-hypertensives, etc.
- Symptoms of hyperandrogenism such as acne, hirsutism, weight gain, and voice change
- *Previous obstetric history*: History of any uterine intervention (e.g. evacuation after a miscarriage or delivery to rule out Asherman's syndrome), infection of the genital tract (e.g. tuberculosis), using intrauterine contraceptive device, etc.
- Symptoms of thyroid dysfunction or Cushing's syndrome.

Marking Scheme

0	1	2	3	4	5	6
Fail		Borderline		Pass		

Likely Differential Diagnosis

- Follicle-stimulating hormone (FSH) levels are significantly raised, which suggest premature ovarian failure. Measurement of FSH and luteinising hormone (LH) levels needs to be repeated after 2 months.[11]
  - This may be related to the past chemotherapy in this patient.
- Hypothalamic cause (psychological stress) would have been the possible cause of her amenorrhoea, had her FSH and LH levels been significantly reduced.

TABLE 7.3: Various causes of secondary amenorrhoea.

No features of androgen excess are present	Features of androgen excess
• Physiological, e.g. pregnancy, lactation, and menopause • Iatrogenic, e.g. depot medroxyprogesterone acetate, contraceptive injection, radiotherapy, and chemotherapy • Systemic disease, e.g. chronic illness, hypo- or hyperthyroidism • Uterine causes, e.g. cervical stenosis and Asherman's syndrome • Ovarian causes, e.g. premature ovarian failure and resistant ovary syndrome • Hypothalamic causes, e.g. weight loss, exercise, psychological distress, chronic illness, and idiopathic • Pituitary causes, e.g. hyperprolactinaemia, hypopituitarism, and Sheehan's syndrome • Hypothalamic/pituitary damage, e.g. tumours, cranial irradiation, head injuries, sarcoidosis, and tuberculosis	• Polycystic ovary syndrome • Cushing's syndrome • Late-onset congenital adrenal hyperplasia • Adrenal or ovarian androgen-producing tumour

- Pregnancy test needs to be done to rule out the presence of pregnancy.
- Measurement of serum TSH and prolactin levels may be required, if symptoms are suggestive of thyroid dysfunction or galactorrhoea, respectively.
- Diagnosis of polycystic ovary syndrome (PCOS) needs to be excluded.
- Progestin challenge test: If the patient bleeds following the administration of exogenous progestins, the diagnosis of anovulation can be established.
- Need for exclusion of other endocrinological causes.
- Various causes of secondary amenorrhoea, which can be encountered in a patient, are enlisted in Table 7.3.[12]

Marking Scheme

0	1	2	3	4	5	6
Fail		Borderline		Pass		

Discussion of an Appropriate Management Plan

- *Implications for her fertility*:
  - Problems related to fertility may affect her relationship with her husband
  - Advice related to fertility must be given only if the patient asks for it
  - May be unable to conceive without the use of reproductive technology
  - May require assisted conception with ovum donation or surrogacy
  - Adoption can be considered in this case
  - Occasional ovulation may be possible in cases of premature menopause.

- *Short-term problems related to premature menopause*:
  - Symptoms of vaginal dryness: This may interfere with sexual function
  - Hot flushes
  - Problems related with bladder function (e.g. incontinence).
- *Long-term problems related to premature menopause*:
  - Increased risk of osteoporosis: Advice bone densitometry in 2–3 years' time
  - Increased risk of cardiovascular disease.
- Consider the use of HRT or combined oral contraceptive pill (OCP) for prevention of short-term and long-term menopausal symptoms. May require long-term use of HRT.
- Can consider the use of complementary therapy instead of conventional HRT.

Marking Scheme

0	1	2	3	4	5	6
Fail		Borderline		Pass		

Role-player's Score

The role-player can award a maximum of 2 marks to the candidate.

Marking Scheme

0	1	2
Role-player never wants to see candidate again	Role-player prepared to see candidate again	Role-player happy to see candidate again

Total score: /20

DISCUSSION

Issues

In this station taking a complete history is very important because it may help detect the possible causes of the secondary amenorrhoea. Pregnancy should be excluded and for this, elicitation of the symptoms of pregnancy and a sexual history including contraception are important. A history of weight loss either induced by exercise or anorexia will suggest a hypothalamic cause. Similarly, information about stress and a sudden change in her circumstances may also suggest a hypothalamic cause. Hyperprolactinaemia may present with a whitish or milky discharge from the breast or only with amenorrhoea. The patient should be enquired if she is taking any drugs that may cause hyperprolactinaemia, [e.g. Rauwolfia alkaloids (antihypertensive), methyldopa, antipsychotic drugs (phenothiazines), etc.]. History of intake of drugs which may cause secondary amenorrhea, e.g. H2 receptor antagonists, Depo-Provera®, danazol, etc. need to be asked. Symptoms suggestive of hyperandrogenism

Flow chart 7.2: Management plan of a patient with secondary amenorrhoea.

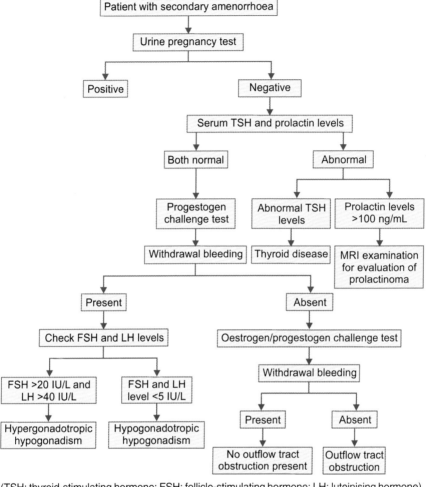

(TSH: thyroid-stimulating hormone; FSH; follicle-stimulating hormone; LH: luteinising hormone)

such as hirsutism, acne, weight gain, voice changes, etc. also need to be asked. This may be suggestive of PCOS or an adrenal tumour. Raised levels of FSH and LH are suggestive of hypergonadotrophic hypogonadism. Though in majority of cases the underlying cause cannot be identified, premature ovarian failure remains an important cause of hypergonadotrophic hypogonadism. In this patient this could be related to her past chemotherapy. If she has had a surgical treatment of a miscarriage or surgical management of postpartum haemorrhage, termination or myomectomy, then Asherman's syndrome must be considered a possibility. Finally, symptoms of thyroid dysfunction and Cushing's syndrome should be excluded. Management plan of a patient with secondary amenorrhoea is described in Flow chart 7.2.

Investigations must be done with aim of excluding the possible causes and to reach a definite diagnosis. Since the patient belongs to a childbearing age group, a pregnancy test helps in excluding presence of any potential pregnancy. A baseline hormone profile test including serum levels of FSH, LH, prolactin, testosterone, sex hormone-binding globulin, androstenedione, TSH, and free T4 needs to be done. Other investigations to be performed would depend on the suspected cause of the amenorrhoea and include a hysteroscopy or hysterosalpingography to diagnose Asherman's syndrome, ultrasound scan of the pelvis to exclude PCOS, and a CT scan of the brain if a tumour is the suspected cause. Karyotype analysis may be done, especially if premature menopause is suspected to be due to turner's mosaic. If genital tuberculosis is suspected as the cause for secondary amenorrhoea, a tuberculin skin test such as the Mantoux test as well as a chest X-ray must be performed.

Pitfalls

In this station based on the findings at the time of taking history, it is difficult to assign a particular cause for secondary amenorrhea. The candidate should present a likely differential diagnosis and exclude or include various differential diagnoses based on the results of different investigations. An important mistake which a candidate can commit is assuming the problem is ovarian in nature and concentrating their answer only on premature menopause.

Variations

Several variations in this kind of station could include different scenarios where the cause of amenorrhea could be related to various causes (Table 7.3).

OSCE STATION 5: PREMENSTRUAL SYNDROME

Candidate's Instructions

You are about to see Mrs Ann Grant, a 37-year-old woman, who has been referred to your outpatient clinic by her GP. A copy of the referral letter is given below.

> The Surgery
> Saint Mary's Lane
> York YO30 7DE
> Dear Gynaecologist
> Re: Mrs Ann Grant, aged 37 years
> I would be very much obliged if you see this patient who has compelled me to refer her for a gynaecological opinion. She says that she has severe premenstrual symptoms, which does not respond to the treatment which I have prescribed her.
> Many thanks.
>
> Yours sincerely
> Dr A Brown (MRCGP)

The task is for 12 minutes (inclusive of 2 minutes of reading time). You have 10 minutes to counsel her about the situation. You shall be awarded marks for the following tasks:

Candidate's tasks:

- Take the relevant history from the patient
- Address the patient's concerns
- Devise an appropriate management plan.

These tasks cover the domains as discussed next.

Core Clinical Skills Domains

Core clinical skills domains tested:

- Patient safety
- Communication with patients
- Information gathering
- Application of knowledge.

Module Tested

The module tested in this station is Module 11 or 'Sexual and Reproductive Health'.

Role-player's Brief

- You are Mrs Ann Grant, 37 years old, assistant to a lawyer and you are extremely unhappy due to the terrible symptoms, which you experience prior to your periods every month. You have consulted your GP several times and he prescribed you some medicines which do not seem to work. Besides some odd vitamins, he also prescribed you OCPs. You used them for 1 month. However, it did not seem to improve your symptoms so you stopped using it. Eventually when your symptoms became unbearable, you urged your GP to refer you to a gynaecologist.
- The symptoms which you often experience include breast tenderness, fluid retention, irritability, emotional outbursts, mood swings, depression, lassitude, insomnia, and sometimes violent behaviour. You feel you are perfectly fine during most days of the month. However, a week prior to your periods, you become extremely irritable and you feel you become a completely different person. You have hit your husband several times during your violent outbursts. As a result, you had been facing marital problems because your partner is extremely vexed with your behaviour.
- You have never faced any psychiatric problems in the past. You were occasionally prescribed a sleeping pill by your GP when you had trouble falling asleep past few years back.
- You tried some over-the-counter preparations including evening primrose oil and some vitamin preparations for premenstrual syndrome (PMS) but that is really not helping you with your symptoms and you have become extremely frustrated with the situation.
- You work as an assistant to a lawyer having a very busy law practice. You find it extremely stressful to deal with your symptoms because the law practice is very busy. You have to frequently meet the clients, be sweet and nice to

them and often offer them counselling. All this becomes very difficult for you because you feel that your personality is not under your control. Your boss often gets upset with you and shouts at you because his practice as well his income suffers because of you. He has asked you to look for another job if you cannot improve your symptoms.

- You first had your periods at the age of 12 years. Since then you have been having regular periods lasting for 4–5 days. Prior to your marriage you rarely experienced premenstrual symptoms of such severe intensity. You experienced some breast tenderness and abdominal cramps prior to your periods.
- You got married 5 years back. Almost since that time, the symptoms you experience prior to your periods have increased in intensity. However, since past 1–2 years the symptoms have become very severe in intensity.
- You do not have any child from your marriage. You however have a 3 years old step son from your husband's previous marriage. He is often the cause of conflict between you and your husband resulting in much stress to you. You yourself had an unwanted pregnancy due to failure of contraception 2 years ago and underwent a surgical termination of the pregnancy. You are currently using condoms for contraception.
- There is no significant medical or surgical history in the past.
- You do not take any medication of note. There is no history of allergies.
- You occasionally smoke cigarettes and drink about 20 units of alcohol per week.
- In your late teens, you had occasionally enjoyed marijuana joint or smoked cocaine once or twice a month. However since then you have not been consuming any recreational drugs.
- Your sister suffered from severe depression and was prescribed anti-depressants for some years.

Prompt Questions
- What disorder am I suffering from?
- Do I have some psychiatric illness?
- What investigations would I require?
- Will I ever get treated?

EXAMINER'S INSTRUCTIONS AND STRUCTURED MARK SHEET

The examiner will mark the candidate on the basis of various tasks which are allotted to the candidate. Out of a total score of 20, the examiner can award a maximum of 18 marks, which are distributed between various candidate tasks as shown next. The role-player can award a maximum of 2 marks to the candidate. Each candidate task must be globally scored by the examiner.

Taking the Relevant History from the Patient

- The candidate needs to elicit the actual symptoms which the patients are experiencing.

- Relation of the symptoms with the timing of the periods needs to be correlated.
- It is important for the candidate to confirm from the patient that the symptoms are definitely premenstrual and disappear by the end of the periods.
- The diagnosis must be confirmed by asking the patient to maintain a symptom diary/calendar or chart.
- Elicit the history regarding the effect of her symptoms on her family life as well as her career.
- Any psychiatric illnesses in the past and any family history of psychiatric illness need to be elicited.
- Any treatments that have been tried previously (both by herself as well as the GP) need to be enquired.

Marking Scheme

0	1	2	3	4	5	6
Fail		Borderline		Pass		

Addressing the Patient's Concerns

- The patient must be explained that if her symptoms are related to the menstrual cycle, she is most likely suffering from premenstrual disorder. In case her symptoms are not related to her menstrual periods, she could be suffering from some other condition.
- She must be counselled that no relevant investigations are required for reaching the diagnosis except that she should maintain a diary for noting down her symptoms in relation to her menstrual periods.
- Though there does not appear to be an underlying psychiatric illness, she would be treated by a multidisciplinary team, involving both gynaecologists and psychologists or psychiatrists.

Marking Scheme

0	1	2	3	4	5	6
Fail		Borderline		Pass		

Devising a Management Plan

- Once the diagnosis of PMS is confirmed, there is a requirement for a multidisciplinary team approach involving gynaecologists, psychologists or psychiatrists wherever it is deemed necessary.
- Various strategies for management of PMS are described in Flow chart 7.3.
- The doctor must emphasise to the patient that many treatments are aimed at suppressing the ovulatory cycle, e.g. combined OCP; progestogens; oestrogens (patches or implants with or without cyclical progestogens); GnRH analogues, etc.

- A therapeutic trial with a GnRH analogue maybe precise and effective for confirming the diagnosis. Response to GnRH therapy is also an indicator that oophorectomy would be successful in that patient.
- Order of the various treatment strategies, which can be adopted include the following (Flow chart 7.3):
  - Counselling/education/reassurance/stress management and relaxation techniques
  - Non-hormonal treatment strategies such as evening primrose oil, vitamin E, pyridoxine, essential fatty acids, etc.—these treatment options may be associated with unpredictable efficacy
  - Selective serotonin reuptake inhibitors (SSRIs) and/or psychotherapy (cognitive behavioural therapy): SSRIs such as fluoxetine can be used in the dosage of 20 or 60 mg.

    Daily treatment with fluoxetine in this case is likely to significantly improve physical symptoms such as breast tenderness, bloating, and headache in women with severe premenstrual syndrome.[13] Physical and psychological symptoms of PMS also improve with SSRIs.

Flow chart 7.3: Management of premenstrual syndrome.

Management of PMS

Mild

First-line therapy:
- Diet and lifestyle changes such as restriction of sodium and caffeine, stress reduction, maintenance of a system diary, exercise, meditation, yoga, CBT
- Counselling, education/reassurance
- Low-dose SSRIs
- Pyridoxine supplements/evening primrose oil, OCPs (Yasmin, cilest)—cyclically or continuously

Moderate

Second-line therapy:
- Oestradiol patches or implants with or without cyclical progestogens
- Progestogens (dihydrogesterone) 20 mg/day, oral medroxyprogesterone acetate 10–30 mg/day or depot medroxyprogesterone acetate 150 mg IM 3 monthly or LNG-IUS
- High-dose SSRIs in the luteal phase

Severe

Third-line therapy:
- GnRH analogues with or without add-back therapy (continuous combined oestrogen + progestogen or tibolone)

Extreme

Fourth-line therapy:
- Total abdominal hysterectomy with bilateral salpingo-oophorectomy with or without HRT (including testosterone)

(CBT: cognitive behavioural therapy; LNG-IUS: levonorgestrel-intrauterine system; SSRIs: selective serotonin reuptake inhibitors; OCPs: oral contraceptive pills; GnRH: gonadotropin-releasing hormone; HRT: hormone replacement therapy; PMS: premenstrual syndrome)

- Oral contraceptive pill/progesterone/danazol
- Oestradiol patches (or implants) plus cyclical progesterone
- Gonadotropin-releasing hormone analogues ± back therapy
- Total abdominal hysterectomy (TAH) and bilateral salpingo-oophorectomy followed by oestrogen HRT.

- Pros and cons of various treatment strategies must be discussed in a non-confrontational and empathic way.
- A clear management strategy including an appropriate and agreed upon follow-up plan must be established in consultation with the patient.

Marking Scheme

0	1	2	3	4	5	6
Fail		Borderline		Pass		

Role-player's Score

The role-player can award a maximum of 2 marks to the candidate.

Marking Scheme

0	1	2
Role-player never wants to see candidate again	Role-player prepared to see candidate again	Role-player happy to see candidate again

Total score: /20

DISCUSSION

Issues

Premenstrual syndrome is common at the extremes of reproductive life. There is no investigation which can be done to establish the diagnosis of premenstrual syndrome. Diagnosis is established with help of accurate history taking. This station tests the candidate's ability to take proper history so as to reach the diagnosis of PMS and to address her concerns regarding this condition. Various treatment options for PMS are available, some of which have a high placebo effect. The treatment prescribed by the doctor is influenced by the factors such as patient's desire for contraception or contraindications to the various options. The first-line non-hormonal treatment regimen involves the use of treatment options such as evening primrose oil, vitamin E, and pyridoxine. Though these treatment options may sometimes help in alleviation of symptoms, the efficacy of these non-hormonal regimens largely remains unpredictable. Psychotherapy in form of cognitive behavioural therapy may also sometimes prove to be helpful. In the absence of contraindications, the combined OCP can be considered as the drug of first choice because it acts by supressing ovulation. The combined OCP may help in providing complete relief against the symptoms or they may limit these symptoms to 1–2 days premenstrually, or they may completely prove to be ineffective.

The second-line therapy comprising the use of oestradiol patches or implants with or without cyclical progestogens help in providing relief against the premenstrual symptoms. Though the use of progestogens helps in reducing the risks of endometrial hyperplasia, this may itself cause premenstrual symptoms and subsequently poor compliance. Combining the oestrogen implants with the levonorgestrel intrauterine contraceptive device is likely to be theoretically associated with fewer systemic side effects, thereby overcoming this problem. However, this option should only be considered if her PMS is very severe and other options have failed. Use of progestogens only may also help in improving symptoms in some patients. Progestogens may be prescribed in the form of tablets or pessaries during the second half of the menstrual cycle. Monthly or 3-monthly progestogen injections (depot medroxyprogesterone acetate or DPMA) may also prove to be effective. Presently, there is insufficient evidence to recommend the routine use of progesterone or progestogens for treatment of PMS symptoms. The use of progesterone or progestogens has not been found to be better than placebo for alleviation of symptoms related to PMS.[14,15]

The third-line therapy for PMS comprises of using GnRH analogues. This may serve as an effective medical option for some patients. They suppress ovarian activity by downregulating the pituitary gland. Use of GnRH analogues not only helps in relieving the symptoms but they may also help in determining if the woman's symptoms are of ovarian or endocrine origin. This information would be helpful in deciding if she would benefit from bilateral oophorectomy. This is a radical but an effective procedure which may require the use of oestrogen HRT as an add-back therapy to help alleviate the occurrence of menopausal symptoms. If this combination is effective, use of therapy may be prolonged beyond 6 months.

More recent therapeutic regimen for premenstrual symptoms includes the use of SSRIs. The use of SSRIs, such as clomipramine and fluoxetine, has been shown to be effective in some patients who experience premenstrual symptoms due to altered serotonergic function.

When treating women with PMS, it is recommended that SSRI therapy should be withdrawn gradually and tapered over a few weeks to avoid withdrawal symptoms, which may occur, if SSRIs have been administered continuously. Abrupt withdrawal of an SSRI may result in side effects such as gastrointestinal disturbances, headache, anxiety, dizziness, paraesthesia, sleep disturbances, fatigue, influenza-like symptoms, sweating, etc.[16]

Non-SSRI antidepressants and anxiolytics have also been shown to improve one or more of the premenstrual symptoms. However, a significant number of women discontinue this treatment due to the presence of unwanted side effects such as drowsiness, nausea, anxiety, and headaches. Nevertheless, psychotherapy (in form of cognitive behavioural therapy) in combination with these drugs may be associated with better results.

Pitfalls

The most important mistake which the candidate can commit on such kinds of stations is offering treatment before confirming the diagnosis. In the first step the candidate must take a complete history to reach the diagnosis of premenstrual syndrome. Physical examination and investigations (such as hormone profile or ultrasound examination) may be required in some cases to confirm the diagnosis. PMS may be sometimes associated with pathologies such as large uterine fibroids, pelvic inflammatory disease, and endometriosis. These need to be elicited at the time of taking history. Moreover, the candidates should avoid using ambiguous phrases, such as 'various treatment options can be tried'.

Variations

Besides premenstrual syndrome, dysmenorrhea (both primary and secondary) is another condition in which taking proper history is important for reaching the correct diagnosis. There could be an OSCE station pertaining to this situation.

REFERENCES

1. Deveugele M, Derese A, De Bacquer D, et al. Consultation in general practice: a standard operating procedure? Patient Educ Couns. 2004;54(2):227-33.
2. General Medical Council. Good medical practice. General medical council: Manchester; 2013.
3. Sankaran S, Manyonda IT. Medical management of fibroids. Best Pract Res Clin Obstet Gynaecol. 2008;22(4):655-76.
4. Taylor DK, Leppert PC. Treatment for Uterine Fibroids: Searching for Effective Drug Therapies. Drug Discov Today Ther Strateg. 2012;9(1):e41-e49.
5. Hackshaw AW, Law MR, Wald NJ. The accumulated evidence on lung cancer and environmental tobacco smoke. BMJ. 1997;315(7114):980-8.
6. Cook DG, Strachan DP. Health effects of passive smoking-10: summary of effects of parental smoking on the respiratory health of children and implications for research. Thorax. 1999;54(4):357-66.
7. Anderson ME, Johnson DC, Batal HA. Sudden infant death syndrome and prenatal maternal smoking: rising attributed risk in the back to sleep era. BMC Med. 2005;11:3-4.
8. Ness RB, Grisso JA, Hirschinger N, et al. Cocaine and tobacco use and the risk of spontaneous abortion. N Engl J Med. 1999;340(5):333-9.
9. National Institute of Clinical Excellence. (2010). Smoking: stopping in pregnancy and after childbirth: public health guideline [PH26]. [online] NICE website. Available from www. nice.org.uk/guidance/ph26 [Accessed September 2017].
10. Royal College of Obstetricians and Gynaecologists. Air travel and pregnancy. RCOG: London; 2015.
11. Goswami D, Conway GS. Premature ovarian failure. Hum Reprod Update. 2005;11:391-410.
12. Maruthini D, Balen A. Modern management of amenorrhoea. Trends in Urology, Gynaecology & Sexual Health, Volume 13, Issue 2, Version of Record online: 17 APR 2008.

13. Steiner M, Romano SJ, Babcock S, et al. The efficacy of fluoxetine in improving physical symptoms associated with premenstrual dysphoric disorder. BJOG. 2001;108(5):462-8.

14. Wyatt K, Dimmock P, Jones P, et al. Efficacy of progesterone and progestogens in management of premenstrual syndrome: systematic review. BMJ. 2001;323(7316): 776-80.

15. Ford O, Lethaby A, Mol BW, et al. Progesterone for premenstrual syndrome. Cochrane Database Syst Rev. 2009;(2):CD003415.

16. Dimmock PW, Wyatt KM, Jones PW, et al. Efficacy of selective serotonin-reuptake inhibitors in premenstrual syndrome: a systematic review. Lancet. 2000;356(9236):1131-6.

CHAPTER

8

Application of Knowledge

INTRODUCTION

The stations which test the candidate's ability to apply clinical knowledge may test the candidate's clinical skills as well as their ability to manage various obstetric or gynaecological problems in the clinics.

CLINICAL SKILLS

The stations testing clinical knowledge usually test the skills which an ST5 level would be commonly performing in the wards, clinics or the operating theatre. These situations usually simulate the scenarios commonly encountered in the clinical practice. In order to perform well at these kinds of stations, the candidates need to mentally imagine themselves to be at the clinic and perform the duties which they would normally have in such kind of scenarios. Some such stations testing the candidate's clinical knowledge may require the candidate to demonstrate some skills (e.g. conducting a vacuum or forceps delivery or a breech vaginal delivery or demonstrating the manoeuvres for management of shoulder dystocia using a manikin). Sometimes such stations could also require the candidate to teach a role-player certain clinical skills.

CLINICAL MANAGEMENT OF GYNAECOLOGICAL OR OBSTETRIC PROBLEMS

In these stations, the candidates may be faced with a scenario in the clinic or the operating theatre or the labour ward and they would be expected to describe how they would manage such situation. The candidates may also be required to interpret the results of various investigations or clinical examination which they may be provided in context of a particular OSCE station.

OSCE STATION 1: DELAYED LABOUR DUE TO OCCIPITOPOSTERIOR POSITION

Candidate's Instructions

Mrs Mitchell Brown, a 32-year-old second gravida, has presented in spontaneous labour at 41 weeks of gestation. On abdominal examination, there is a single live foetus in longitudinal lie, cephalic presentation. The foetal head is still two-fifths palpable per abdomen. She is experiencing contractions at the rate of 2–3 every 15–20 minutes, with the contractions lasting for 20–25 seconds. Vaginal examination shows the cervix to be 3–4 cm dilated and fully effaced. Foetal head is at –1 (minus 1 station). Caput is present. The occiput is present posteriorly on the right side. She had spontaneous rupture of her membranes 5–6 hours ago and was 3 cm dilated at that stage. A midwife has asked you to review the case and agree to a management plan with Mitchell. The task is for 12 minutes (inclusive of 2 minutes of reading time). You have 10 minutes to counsel her about the situation. You shall be awarded marks for the following tasks:

> **Candidate's tasks:**
> - Take a relevant history from the patient to establish the complete extent of the situation
> - Agree to a management plan taking into account the patient's wishes
> - Advice regarding the immediate steps to be taken in this case.
> *Three hours later her pain gets much worse and the cardiotocography (CTG) is suspicious. On vaginal examination, the cervix was found to be fully dilated with the head in occipitoposterior position 2 cm below the ischial spines.*
> - What would your subsequent management be?

These tasks cover the domains as discussed next.

Core Clinical Skills Domains

> **Core clinical skills domains tested:**
> - Patient safety
> - Communication with patients
> - Information gathering
> - Application of knowledge.

Module Tested

The module tested in this station is Module 6 or 'Management of Labour'.

Role-player's Brief

You are Mrs Mitchell Brown, a 32-year-old patient and you are pregnant with your second child. This was a planned pregnancy, which has reached 41 weeks. Your first child, Ann is 5-year-old girl. You were booked in the maternity unit at 10 weeks. All the blood tests and ultrasound examinations performed in the antenatal period were found to be within normal limits. You have your dating ultrasound records, according to which you are 41 weeks of gestation. Your antenatal period had largely been uneventful and you enjoyed your pregnancy. Antenatal care has been provided by your midwife as you do not like hospitals. Your previous delivery was at a midwifery-led unit (MLU) and you prefer that this time as well.

You will be simulating a strong contraction while the doctor is talking to you. If the doctor does not pause, while you are simulating the contraction, you must make it clear that you are in pain and you do not understand what the doctor is talking about.

You and your partner Jake have done an extensive research on internet regarding labour and childbirth and are very keen for minimal intervention. You want to have a natural childbirth as far as possible. You do not mind intermittent monitoring of the baby's heartbeat but you are adamant against continuous CTG monitoring. Ideally, you want a water birth in the MLU and you are extremely scared about application of instruments to deliver your baby. During your second trimester ultrasound, you were informed that you are carrying a baby boy. You have named this boy as Louis. You are also extremely concerned about bonding with Louis and breastfeeding him. Overall the well-being of Louis is extremely important for you. In case there is a threat to the baby, you are willing to be flexible if the doctor proposes a sensible management plan to you in the interests of your baby. The doctor may advice you to get transferred to the consultant-led labour ward for continuous CTG monitoring and application of ventouse. The doctor may tell you that your baby's head is positioned in such a way that it might delay the baby's birth. There is a possibility that baby delivers on its own. However, in some cases there is need to facilitate the baby's delivery through application of instruments; for example, vacuum or forceps. You are completely against the plan of transfer to a consultant led unit. However, you would agree to a compromise such as transfer to the labour ward and CTG monitoring alone. After some time of monitoring, the doctor would explain to you that that the baby's heart trace (CTG) is showing some abnormality which is not dangerous at the moment, but the baby's delivery needs to be expedited with help of vacuum or forceps application to ensure the baby's well-being.

Prompt Questions

- Doctor I do not want continuous monitoring of my baby with the help of machines. Is this possible?
- Can I not have a water birth with the help of midwifes?
- Is it not possible to deliver Louis without the application of instruments?
- I do not want Louis delivered by the consultants. Can you please help me with this?

EXAMINER'S INSTRUCTIONS AND STRUCTURED MARK SHEET

The examiner will mark the candidate on the basis of various tasks which are allotted to the candidate. Out of a total score of 20, the examiner can award a maximum of 18 marks, which are distributed between various candidate tasks as shown next. The role-player can award a maximum of 2 marks to the candidate. Each candidate task must be globally scored by the examiner.

Taking a Relevant History from the Patient to Establish the Complete Extent of the Situation

- Establishes the full extent of the situation, including the patient's wishes.
- The wordings of the question, 'establish the complete extent' should give the candidate a clue that there is more to this scenario than just managing primary arrest in labour with occipitoposterior position.
- A relevant obstetric history must be taken by the candidate.
- Role player's views regarding labour and delivery must be ascertained.
- Enquire about 'the role-player's wishes' as well as her clinical background.
- The candidate must ask open questions related to the patient's concerns and determine the reasons for her concerns. The candidates must encourage the role-player to share with them her desire for a natural birth with no intervention.
- A competent candidate would explain the situation using simple language, avoiding the use of medical terminology, e.g. occipitoposterior position, latent phase, and significance of lack of progress.
- A competent candidate would personalise discussion, pause while the patient is having a contraction and asks her if it is alright to carry on after the contraction is over.
- The role-player must be explained that the current situation may be placing her baby at an increased risk and so necessary action may be required in order to prevent harm to the baby.
- Delay in progress of labour due to occipitoposterior position must be explained.
- The abnormality in foetal heart must be recognised, and expediting delivery with vacuum application be advised.
- She should be advised to get admitted in the obstetric labour ward for intermittent CTG monitoring.
- The competent candidate must adopt a nonthreatening style, recognizing the patient's plan for her labour experience.

Marking Scheme

0	1	2	3	4	5
Fail		Borderline		Pass	

Agreeing to a Management Plan Taking into Account the Patient's Wishes

- A competent candidate would reach a compromise with the role-player and agree to a management plan.

- The role-player would be reassured that nothing will be done without her consent, while ensuring that she is able to understand the probable hazards and repercussions of noncompliance.
- The candidate must lay emphasis on the advice for increased monitoring and involvement of consultant in her care. She must be advised regarding the requirement for transfer to the obstetric labour ward for additional care.
- A competent candidate would explain the role-player about the requirement to inform the consultant.
- In case, the patient does not agree upon a management plan, she should be advised of the risks involved. A mutually agreed-upon management plan must be negotiated with the role-player to keep the mother and baby as safe as possible.

Marking Scheme

0	1	2	3	4	5	6
Fail		Borderline		Pass		

Immediate Management Plan

- Shifting the role-player to an obstetric labour unit
- Negotiating a plan for intermittent CTG monitoring.

Marking Scheme

0	1	2	3
Fail		Borderline	Pass

Three hours later her pain gets much worse and the CTG trace shows suspicious changes on CTG. She was found on examination to be fully dilated with the head occipitoposterior, 2 cm below the ischial spines. What would be your subsequent management plan?

Subsequent Management Plan

- Explain her about the urgency of the situation without alarming her.
- Explain about the requirement for forceps or ventouse application.

Marking Scheme

0	1	2	3	4
Fail		Borderline		Pass

Role-player's Score

The role-player can award a maximum of 2 marks to the candidate.

Marking Scheme

0	1	2
Role-player never wants to see candidate again	Role-player prepared to see candidate again	Role-player happy to see candidate again

Total score: /20

DISCUSSION

Issues

This scenario tests the candidate's core knowledge. This situation, of slow progress labour in a primigravida due to occipitoposterior position, is commonly encountered by the ST5 trainees in clinical practice. The main thing which this station assesses is the candidate's ability for engaging in the shared decision making.[1] The candidates must carefully read wordings of the allocated tasks. Use of the word 'agree' rather than 'decide on' should give them a clue that the role-player is likely to disagree with the standard advice. This station, therefore, tests the candidate's skills of being able to negotiate with the patient while ensuring not only her safety, but also that of the baby. The candidate must be able to establish a good rapport with the role-player. They must also be able to diplomatically deal with her unwillingness to accept their advice without getting angry or arguing and shouting at her. The actor has been briefed to agree to a compromise if approached properly by the candidate. The task is clearly assessing the patient's safety. At the same time it is important for the candidate to be able to clearly maintain a balance between elements of patient safety and agreement with a patient's request which may put herself or her baby at risk.

Pitfalls

The station mainly tests the candidate's ability to reach a mutually agreed upon management plan with the role-player. Forcing the role-player to agree upon a management plan can be considered as a potential mistake. Instructing the patient to move to the consultant-led labour ward, forcing her to get her baby delivered using instrument delivery (vacuum or forceps), without taking into account the patient's wishes can be considered as an important mistake in this kind of station. Bullying, threatening her, and frightening her by continuously talking about the seriousness of the situation are other pitfalls which the candidates must avoid.

Variations

The different kinds of scenarios possible with this kind of station include the patients in different stages of labour; there could be nonprogress or normal progress; there could be superimposed clinical condition (e.g. meconium-stained liquor or pathological CTG) requiring expedited delivery.

Superimposed on this scenario, there could be a situation where the role-player refuses for any intervention or wants to wait for her husband.

OSCE STATION 2: PREMATURE LABOUR

Candidate's Instructions

The patient you are about to see is Miss Sofia James and she has just been admitted to your maternity unit. The midwife has examined her and is concerned. Her period of gestation is 30 weeks and appears to be having uterine contractions. You are the registrar on duty posted in the labour ward and so the midwife seeks your help. She asks you to assess Mrs James.

Her examination reveals the following findings:

- Temperature: 37°C
- Blood pressure: 130/80 mmHg
- Pulse rate: 90 beats/min
- Abdominal palpation: Single live foetus is breech presentation corresponding to 30 weeks of gestation. The uterus appears irritable. However, there is no uterine tenderness.
- Vaginal examination: The cervix is slightly effaced, and 1–2 cm dilated. Presenting part is at the level of spines and the membranes are intact.

The task is for 12 minutes (inclusive of 2 minutes of reading time). You have 10 minutes to counsel her about the situation. You shall be awarded marks for the following tasks:

> **Candidate's tasks:**
> - Take a relevant obstetric history
> - What are the probable differential diagnoses?
> - What relevant investigations would you like to order?
> - Formulate an appropriate management plan.

These tasks cover the domains as discussed next.

Core Clinical Skills Domains

> **Core clinical skills domains tested:**
> - Communication with patients
> - Information gathering
> - Application of knowledge.

Module Tested

The module tested in this station is Module 6 or 'Management of Labour'.

Role-player's Brief

- You are Miss Sofia James, 22-year-old woman.
- Your present pregnancy is your second one and presently you have reached 30 weeks of gestation.

- Your previous pregnancy was 5 years back as a teenager and had resulted due to a one-night stand you had while you were in college. You had got this pregnancy aborted at 8 weeks of gestation.
- This present pregnancy is unplanned and is the outcome of the relationship with your boyfriend, resulting due to failed barrier contraception.
- Your LMP was 30 weeks back (LMP = date of examination – 30 weeks).
- EDD is after 10 weeks (EDD = date of examination + 10 weeks).
- Initially you were not sure if you wanted to keep this baby. Eventually your boyfriend convinced you to keep the baby. You agreed with reluctance. Presently you have an indifferent attitude towards your pregnancy.
- You booked in the maternity unit at 16 weeks.
- All the antenatal blood tests and ultrasound scans have been normal so far.
- Antenatal care has been provided by your midwife as you do not like to visit the hospital.
- An ultrasound scan done during the first few weeks of pregnancy showed a normally grown foetus equivalent to your dates.
- The morning before admission you had felt generally unwell and developed intermittent abdominal cramps, somewhat resembling menstrual cramps. With the progress of the day, the abdominal pains became more regular and had taken the nature of uterine contractions. When you decided to go to the hospital, the pain was coming after an interval of every 4–5 minutes and was lasting for 30–45 seconds. You have also had some mucoid, blood-stained vaginal discharge. You, however, did not experience frank bleeding or passage of clear water per vaginam (suggesting that your waters have broken).
- You are single, unemployed and live at home with your parents, three sisters, and two brothers. You get along very well with all your siblings.
- Family history: Your mother has type 2 diabetes, which is controlled with help of medicines.
- You smoke about 5–10 cigarettes a day, and drink alcohol at the weekends (6–7 bottles of beer). You do not do drugs.
- You are presently not sure what you are going to do regarding your accommodation when the baby arrives. You would probably move in your boyfriend's apartment, you still need to talk to him.
- You underwent an appendectomy when you were 12 years old.
- You were diagnosed with mild asthma since you were 5 years old and occasionally require the use of Ventolin® inhaler for asthma when essential but not on a regular basis.
- Besides this, there is no significant treatment history and there is no history of any allergies.

Prompt Questions

- What is the cause of my pain?
- Is this a sign that I am about to deliver?

EXAMINER'S INSTRUCTIONS AND STRUCTURED MARK SHEET

The examiner will mark the candidate on the basis of various tasks which are allotted to the candidate. Out of a total score of 20, the examiner can award a maximum of 18 marks, which are distributed between various candidate tasks as shown next. The role-player can award a maximum of 2 marks to the candidate. Each candidate task must be globally scored by the examiner.

History Taking

- History regarding the presenting complaints:
  - Nature of her abdominal pain (constant or comes and goes?)
  - Does the pain radiate? (If yes, where does the pain radiate to?)
  - Any precipitating factors
  - If pain resembling uterine contractions: Sequence and timing of these contractions
  - Presence of back pain or pelvic pressure.
- History of any discharge or bleeding, or loss of liquor via vagina
- History suggestive of any underlying infection: Burning micturition, fever, bowel problems, etc.
- History suggestive of abruption: History of abdominal trauma, pre-eclampsia, cocaine abuse, reduced foetal movements, vaginal bleeding, etc.
- History of current pregnancy:
  - LMP or EDD
  - Planned or unplanned pregnancy
  - Type of antenatal care she has received
  - Results of the blood tests or ultrasound scan during the antenatal period
  - Presence of any other complaints or complications during the antenatal period.
- Other history:
  - Obstetric history (history regarding previous pregnancies)
  - Social history (history related to smoking cigarette, alcohol intake, and recreational drug use)
  - Relevant family history
  - Relevant past medical or surgical history
  - Previous history of any previous sexually transmitted diseases.

Marking Scheme

0	1	2	3	4	5
Fail		Borderline		Pass	

Differential Diagnosis

- Preterm labour appears to be the most likely diagnosis
- Other differential diagnoses include urinary tract infection (UTI), concealed abruption or bowel problems.

Marking Scheme

0	1	2	3
Fail		Borderline	Pass

Investigations

Various investigations which need to be done include the following described next.

Investigations for Ruling Out Infection

- Sending the midstream urine (MSU) sample for routine and microscopy
- Full blood count
- C-reactive protein.

Confirming the Presence of Preterm Labour[2]

Uterine activity monitoring: Hospital based external CTG has been found to be effective in monitoring of uterine contractions for evaluating preterm labour.

Fibronectin test: A cutoff value of 50 ng/mL is considered positive and highly predictive of preterm labour.

Transvaginal ultrasound: Transvaginal ultrasound examination is required for confirming the foetal size and presentation, measurement of cervical length, funnelling of cervical canal, presence of any retroplacental clot, and foetal well-being.

Marking Scheme

0	1	2	3	4
Fail		Borderline		Pass

Management Plan

- Patient needs to be admitted to the labour ward for close monitoring of uterine contractions and initiating treatment for prolonging the pregnancy.
- Use of tocolytic agents to inhibit the uterine contractions (use of ritodrine or atosiban according to the department protocol).
- Administration of intramuscular steroids for promoting foetal pulmonary maturity, thereby, reducing the severity of respiratory distress syndrome.[3]
- Deciding the mode of delivery in view of breech presentation in case the patient goes into labour.
- Foetal surveillance and monitoring: Careful monitoring of the preterm foetus preferably by continuous electronic monitoring for signs of foetal hypoxia and acidosis.
- Prophylactic therapy for group B streptococcal infection should be administered, especially in the cases where membranes have also ruptured or signs of infection are present.

- In case of anticipated delivery, the paediatrician needs to be informed as the baby may require transfer to a tertiary unit. Availability of the cot in the neonatal intensive care unit needs to be discussed in advance. Delivery must be conducted in presence of an expert neonatologist capable of dealing with the complications of prematurity.

Marking Scheme

0	1	2	3	4	5	6
Fail		Borderline		Pass		

Role-player's Score

The role-player can award a maximum of 2 marks to the candidate.

Marking Scheme

0	1	2
Role-player never wants to see candidate again	Role-player prepared to see candidate again	Role-player happy to see candidate again

Total score: /20

DISCUSSION

Issues

This station particularly tests the candidates' ability to apply their clinical knowledge and take an appropriate history so as to reach the correct diagnosis. The station is directed towards the diagnosis of preterm labour. The candidate needs to demonstrate the ability to reach the diagnosis of preterm labour on the basis of patient's history. He/she should also be able to order relevant investigations which are able to supplement the diagnosis established on taking history.

The clinical presentations suggestive of preterm labour include the following:[4]

- Cervical dilatation of greater than or equal to 1 cm and effacement of 80% or more
- Uterine contractions of greater than or equal to 4 per 20 minutes or greater than or equal to 8 per hour, lasting for more than 40 seconds
- Cervical length on transvaginal ultrasound scan less than or equal to 2.5 cm and funnelling of internal os
- Symptoms such as menstrual cramps, pelvic pressure, backache and/or vaginal discharge or bleeding
- Bishop's score may be 4 or greater
- Lower uterine segment may be thinned out and the presenting part may be deep in the pelvis.

Based on the findings of clinical examination, preterm labour can be of two types:

1. *Early preterm labour*: In cases of early preterm labour, cervical effacement is greater than or equal to 80% and cervical dilatation is greater than or equal to 1 cm, but less than 3 cm.
2. *Advanced preterm labour*: In cases of advanced preterm labour, cervical dilatation is greater than or equal to 3 cm.

Management of preterm labour is described in Flow chart 8.1.

Flow chart 8.1: Management of preterm labour.

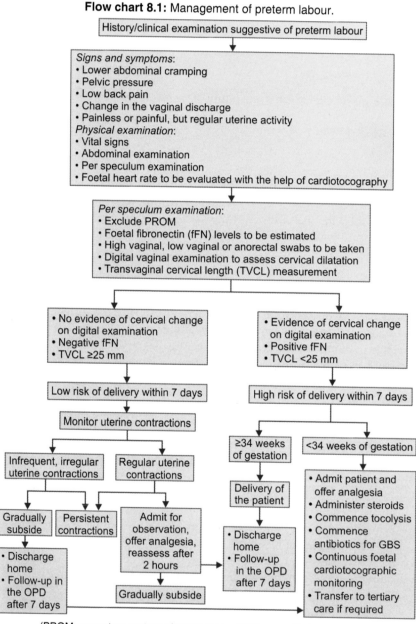

(PROM: premature rupture of membranes; GBS: group B streptococcus)

Pitfalls

A capable candidate would be able to establish a diagnosis of early preterm labour in this case. However, they need to determine if the patient is likely to progress to advanced preterm labour. Failure to order investigations for predicting preterm birth can be considered as an important mistake in this type of station.

Variations

Another variation in this kind of station could be a patient presenting in advanced preterm labour.

OSCE STATION 3: ABNORMAL CARDIOTOCOGRAPHY

Candidate's Instructions

You are the SpR on call and have been called to evaluate a patient, Mrs Sarah Norman, in Room no. 4 of the labour ward. She is a 35-year-old primigravida who is now 14 days past her due date. Besides being post-dated, her antenatal period had largely been uneventful. She had presented to the emergency department with the complaints of reduced foetal movements. Vaginal examination shows a 1-2 cm cervical dilatation and a partially effaced cervix. The foetal presentation is cephalic. The head is fully engaged and is palpated at +1 station. A cardiotocographic trace was taken by her midwife (Fig. 8.1). After seeing the trace, the midwife is extremely worried and therefore she shows the trace to you. The task is for 12 minutes (inclusive of 2 minutes of reading time). You have 10 minutes to counsel her about the situation. You shall be awarded marks for the following tasks:

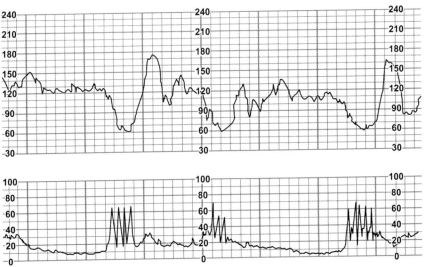

Fig. 8.1: Cardiotocographic trace of Sarah Norman.

Candidate's tasks:

- Discuss the patient's CTG
- Address the patient's concerns
- Discuss further management of her labour.

These tasks cover the domains as discussed next.

Core Clinical Skills Domains

Core clinical skills domains tested:

- Patient safety
- Communication with patients
- Information gathering
- Application of knowledge.

Module Tested

The module tested in this station is Module 6 or 'Management of Labour'.

Role-player's Brief

- You are Mrs Sarah Norman, 35 year old, and you live with your partner who works as a primary schoolteacher.
- This is your first pregnancy and you had been long trying to become pregnant. Thus, this pregnancy is precious for you and you feel you are having the best time in your life. Your antenatal period had largely been uneventful. You have thoroughly enjoyed the period of your pregnancy and share a wonderful relationship with your midwife.
- All this while you had been collaborating with your midwife and did not feel the requirement to meet your consultant. You and your partner had initially wanted a home birth with as little medical intervention as possible. However, your midwife convinced you to have a hospital delivery because she felt that the home delivery might not be best option for the baby as this was your first baby.
- You have had regular antenatal check-ups throughout your pregnancy and all your scans and blood tests have been normal.
- As you reached 40 weeks of gestation, you did not experience any symptom suggestive of labour.
- At 41 weeks of gestation, your midwife advised you to get admitted to get your labour induced. However, you were adamant that you want a natural birth and would not get your labour induced. She took your cardiotocographic trace at that time and assured you about foetal well-being.
- Now you have reached 42 weeks of gestation. You have been extremely frightened since last night because you have been experiencing reduced foetal movements since last evening. Your partner is devoted to you, but he is out of country due to some official work. You have spoken to him. He is planning to take the next flight and reach home as soon as possible. You, however, decide to go to the hospital on your own because you are

really worried about your baby's well-being. You are initially not ready to be monitored, but eventually you get ready to do so for your baby's sake.
- You are concerned about the welfare of your baby and want the doctor to clearly explain you the results of the cardiotocograph trace.

Prompt Questions

- What does my trace show?
- Is there anything to worry about?
- Is my baby alright?

EXAMINER'S INSTRUCTIONS AND STRUCTURED MARK SHEET

The examiner will mark the candidate on the basis of various tasks which are allotted to the candidate. Out of a total score of 20, the examiner can award a maximum of 18 marks, which are distributed between various candidate tasks as shown next. The role-player can award a maximum of 2 marks to the candidate. Each candidate task must be globally scored by the examiner.

Discussion of CTG Trace

- The role-player should be counselled regarding the probable foetal risk due to reduced foetal movements and post-dated pregnancy.
- The pattern of uterine contractions, whether occurring regularly or not, can also be assessed on CTG.
- Four main features of the FHR, which must be observed on the cardiotocograph include the following: (1) baseline heart rate; (2) baseline variability; (3) decelerations; and (4) acceleration. The value of these parameters as observed on the patient's CTG trace are as follows:
  - *Baseline FHR:* Varying between 120 beats/min to 130 beats/min.
  - *Variability:* Variability is normal to reduced
  - *Accelerations:* There are no accelerations
  - *Decelerations:* Deep variable decelerations are present
- *Opinion:* This CTG trace falls into the suspicious category because one of the features (atypical variable decelerations) falls in the non-reassuring category, while remainder of the features are reassuring. Such a trace at such an early stage of labour is worrisome.

Marking Scheme

0	1	2	3	4	5	6
Fail		Borderline		Pass		

Addressing the Patient's Concerns

Concerns about the Foetal Well-being

- The role-player is present in early stage of labour as she is only 1–2 cm dilated. Considering the fact that she may dilate at the rate of 1 cm per hour, she may be in labour for another 8 hours.

- During the early stage of labour, the foetus may be already showing signs of distress on the CTG or may have passed meconium. Therefore, it may be worth rupturing her membranes during this stage.
- Continuous monitoring is required using CTG for monitoring the foetal well-being.
- It would be difficult to do a foetal blood sampling (FBS) at this stage because the cervix is only 1–2 cm dilated. Also, if FBS is done at this stage, it may have to be repeated several times in the future. An option could be to do FBS at a later stage when the cervix is 5–6 cm dilated in case the non-reassuring changes on the CTG persist.
- Possible diagnosis could be cord compression. This could be related to reduced liquor and a large-sized baby as a result of post-dated pregnancy.

Concerns about the Maternal Well-being

- Intravenous (IV) access needs to be established.
- Continuous monitoring of the mother (pulse, BP and temperature) as well as input and output charting.
- Complete blood count along with blood group and save needs to be done in anticipation of an operative delivery.

Marking Scheme

0	1	2	3	4	5	6
Fail		Borderline		Pass		

Discussion Regarding Further Management

- Reveals the urgency of the situation of the patient.
- Negotiates a plan with the patient (Flow chart 8.2): Monitoring with CTG for a few hours if the foetal heart tracing remains non-reassuring. Caesarean delivery would be immediately required if the foetal heart trace becomes pathological anytime in future.
- Consent form needs to be signed:
  - Enquire about the husband, when would he be able to reach the hospital?
  - Take patient's own consent while the husband is away.
- Type of anaesthesia (spinal versus general anaesthesia) needs to be decided.
- Paediatricians need to be present at the time of delivery.
- Availability of a cot in the neonatal unit needs to be checked because there is a possibility that the baby may have to be admitted to the neonatal unit post-delivery.

Marking Scheme

0	1	2	3	4	5	6
Fail		Borderline		Pass		

Flow chart 8.2: Management of post-term pregnancies.

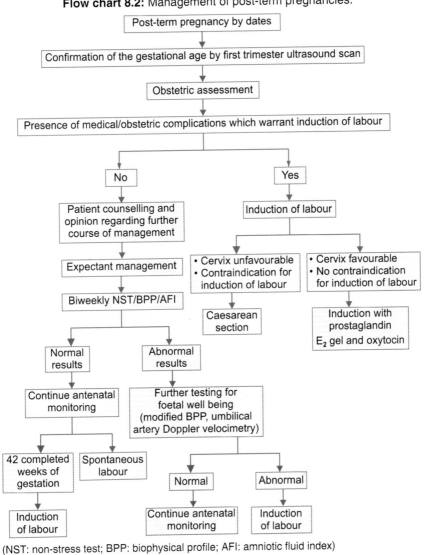

(NST: non-stress test; BPP: biophysical profile; AFI: amniotic fluid index)

Role-player's Score

The role-player can award a maximum of 2 marks to the candidate.

Marking Scheme

0	1	2
Role-player never wants to see candidate again	Role-player prepared to see candidate again	Role-player happy to see candidate again

Total score: /20

DISCUSSION

Issues

This station specifically tests the candidate's ability to interpret the CTG trace. In clinical practice, CTG traces are not evaluated on the basis of individual features. Instead, an overall assessment is made on the basis of a number of features. This is used for making clinical decisions in the light of clinical factors and the stage of labour. Categorisation of FHR traces is described in Table 8.1. This is based on NICE classification of FHR features (Table 8.2), which classifies the cardiotocographic traces as normal, nonreassuring, and abnormal based on the four important characteristics of foetal heart trace, i.e. (1) baseline heart rate, (2) variability, (3) decelerations, and (4) accelerations. Traces classified as 'abnormal' are likely to be associated with an increase in the incidence of neonatal encephalopathy, cerebral palsy, neonatal acidosis, and APGAR score of less than 7 at 5 minutes.

Pitfalls

The candidate must remember to discuss the abnormal CTG trace under four headings: baseline heart rate, baseline variability, presence of decelerations, and accelerations. Failing to discuss the abnormal CTG results under these four headings and abruptly reaching the conclusion that the CTG trace is abnormal is a potential mistake which a candidate can commit.

TABLE 8.1: NICE classification of foetal heart rate features.[5]

Foetal heart rate types	Baseline rate (beats/min)	Variability (beats/min)	Decelerations	Acceleration
Normal	110–160	5 to 25	None or early Variable decelerations with no concerning characteristics* for less than 90 minutes	Present: If repeated accelerations are present with reduced variability, the foetal heart rate trace should be regarded as reassuring
Non-reassuring	100–109[†] or 161–180	Less than 5 for 30 to 50 minutes Or More than 25 for 15 to 25 minutes	Variable decelerations with no concerning characteristics* for 90 minutes or more Or Variable decelerations with any concerning characteristics* in up to 50% of contractions for 30 minutes or more	A foetal tachycardia of 160–180 beats/min, where accelerations are present, but no other adverse feature is present should be regarded as suspicious

Contd...

Contd...

Foetal heart rate types	Baseline rate (beats/min)	Variability (beats/min)	Decelerations	Acceleration
			Or Variable decelerations with any concerning characteristics* in over 50% of contractions for less than 30 minutes Or Late decelerations in over 50% of contractions for less than 30 minutes, with no maternal or foetal clinical risk factors such as vaginal bleeding or significant meconium	Absence of accelerations in an otherwise normal cardiotocography is of uncertain significance
Abnormal	<100 >180 Sinusoidal pattern ≥10 minutes	Less than 5 for more than 50 minutes Or More than 25 for more than 25 minutes Or Sinusoidal pattern ≥10 minutes	*Atypical variable decelerations:* Variable decelerations with any concerning characteristics* in over 50% of contractions for 30 minutes (or less if any maternal or foetal clinical risk factors is present) Or *Late decelerations:* Late decelerations for 30 minutes (or less if any maternal or foetal clinical risk factors) Or *Bradycardia/prolonged deceleration:* Acute bradycardia, or a single prolonged deceleration lasting for 3 minutes or more	

(NICE: National Institute for Health and Care Excellence)
*Characteristics of variable decelerations:
• Lasting more than 60 seconds
• Reduced baseline variability within the deceleration
• Failure to return to baseline
• Biphasic (W) shape
• No shouldering.
†Although a baseline foetal heart rate between 100 beats/min and 109 beats/min is a non-reassuring feature, continue usual care if there is normal baseline variability and no variable or late decelerations.

TABLE 8.2: Management based on interpretation of cardiotocograph traces.[5]

Category	Definition	Management
Normal	All features are reassuring	• Continue CTG monitoring and usual care • Counselling the woman and her birth companion(s) about the situation
Suspicious	1 non-reassuring feature and 2 reassuring features	• Correction of any underlying causes, such as hypotension or uterine hyperstimulation • Performing a full set of maternal observations • Beginning 1 or more conservative measures* • Informing an obstetrician or a senior midwife • Documenting a plan for reviewing the whole clinical picture and the CTG findings • Counselling the woman and her birth companion(s) about the situation and taking their preferences into account

Pathological	1 abnormal feature *or* 2 non-reassuring features	• Obtaining a review by an obstetrician and a senior midwife
		• Exclusion of acute events (e.g. cord prolapse, suspected placental abruption or suspected uterine rupture)
		• Correction of any underlying causes, such as hypotension or uterine hyperstimulation
		• Starting 1 or more conservative measures*
		• Counselling the woman and her birth companion(s) about the situation and taking their preferences into account
		• If the cardiotocograph trace is still pathological after implementing conservative measures, the following need to be done:
		  – Obtaining a further review by an obstetrician and a senior midwife
		  – Offering digital foetal scalp stimulation and documenting the outcome
		  – If the cardiotocograph trace is still pathological after foetal scalp stimulation, foetal blood sampling must be considered
		  – The baby's birth must be expedited taking the woman's preferences into account

Need for urgent intervention	Acute bradycardia, or a single prolonged deceleration for 3 minutes or more	• Urgently seek obstetric help • If there has been an acute event (e.g. cord prolapse, suspected placental abruption or suspected uterine rupture), expedite the baby's birth • Correction of any underlying causes, such as hypotension or uterine hyperstimulation • Starting 1 or more conservative measures* • Make preparations for an urgent birth • Counselling the woman and her birth companion(s) about the situation and taking their preferences into account • Expediting the baby's birth if the acute bradycardia persists for 9 minutes • If the foetal heart rate recovers at any time up to 9 minutes, the decision to expedite the birth must be reassessed in discussion with the woman

(CTG: cardiotocograph)

*If there are any concerns about the baby's well-being, be aware of the possible underlying causes and start one or more of the following conservative measures based on an assessment of the most likely cause(s): encouraging the woman to mobilise or adopt an alternative position (and to avoid being supine); offering intravenous fluids if the woman is hypotensive; reducing the frequency of contraction by reducing or stopping oxytocin if it is being used and/or offering a tocolytic drug (a suggested regimen is subcutaneous terbutaline 0.25 mg).

Source: National Institute of Clinical Excellence. (updated 2017) Intrapartum care for healthy women and babies (CG190). NICE: London.

Variations

Different variations in such kind of stations can include CTG traces showing a wide range of changes, varying from normal to non-reassuring to abnormal.

OSCE STATION 4: RETAINED SWAB

Candidate's Instructions

You are on call for the maternity unit and are about to meet Mrs Michelle Bryant-Smyth, who has presented late in the evening, having delivered her first baby child 2 weeks previously. The task is for 12 minutes (inclusive of 2 minutes of reading time). You have 10 minutes to counsel her about the situation. You shall be awarded marks for the following tasks:

Candidate's tasks:
- Establish the circumstances leading to the patient's attendance
- Counsel the patient about the situation and address her concerns
- Advise on the next steps of management in this patient.

These tasks cover the domains as discussed next.

Core Clinical Skills Domains

Core clinical skills domains tested:
- Patient safety
- Communication with patients
- Information gathering
- Application of knowledge.

Module Tested

The module tested in this station is Module 8 or 'Postpartum Problems (the puerperium).'

Role-player's Brief

You are Michelle Bryant-Smyth, a 35-year-old pharmacist living with Peter Murray, a recruitment consultant. You gave birth to your daughter Sofia 2 weeks ago in the maternity unit under the care of consultant obstetrician Mr Phele. This was your second pregnancy and it appeared uneventful antenatally. You have had a previous full-term normal vaginal delivery. At that time, you had delivered a baby boy, James, who is presently 7 years old.

The present pregnancy was uncomplicated but you had prolonged labour at term. Eventually a normal delivery took place with the help of forceps. The reason which the midwife gave you for application of forceps was a large-sized baby. Sofia weighed more than 4 kg at birth. An episiotomy was also given at the time of forceps application. Following the baby's delivery, the midwife told you that your episiotomy had extended up to your anal sphincter (valve controlling the passage of faeces) and would be required to be stitched. The midwife felt unsure while stitching the cut and so the SpR was also called. It seemed to take a long time for her to complete the process.

Following the repair of your vaginal cut and anal sphincter repair, you were advised to have a liquid diet. You were discharged after 1 day. At the time of discharge, you felt perfectly normal except that there was slight discomfort while passing faeces. You were prescribed some laxatives and antibiotics. You were concerned about the safety of these drugs as you were breastfeeding your baby. However, you were reassured about the safety of these drugs by the midwife.

You were happy to get back home with your little girl child, Sofia. You have been breastfeeding her and she appears to be progressing normally. However, 3–4 days following discharge, discomfort in the vaginal and anal region progressively increased. Since past 2 days, you have been having terrible pain in the vaginal area. You have also felt feverish. This evening while taking a shower you felt as if there was a piece of material in the vaginal area. You were frightened, but you managed to pull out that odd thing. You and your partner inspected the material which was extremely foul smelling and reached the conclusion that probably something had been left in the vagina at the time of repair. You and your partner are extremely angry about what has happened and decide to go to the hospital immediately. You have kept the piece of material in the plastic bag. You feel that the hospital staff has made a mistake and you are worried that if this would have remained inside, it could have caused you further harm. You feel this is negligence on part of the staff and want to file an official complaint. You also want an apology and explanation for the events, which have occurred. The piece of material in the plastic bag is extremely foul smelling and you do not want the plastic bag to be opened. Nor do you want to hand over this piece of evidence to anyone unless you are clearly explained about the reasons. However, you would be ready to do so if the reasons have been clearly explained to you.

Prompt Questions

- Was the person who performed the repair competent enough to be doing so on her own?
- How do you explain that the swab count appeared correct but one was left in my vagina?
- I plan to register a complaint and seek legal advice. Whom do I contact?

EXAMINER'S INSTRUCTIONS AND STRUCTURED MARK SHEET

The examiner will mark the candidate on the basis of various tasks, which are allotted to the candidate. Out of a total score of 20, the examiner can award a maximum of 18 marks, which are distributed between various candidate tasks as shown next. The role-player can award a maximum of 2 marks to the candidate. Each candidate task must be globally scored by the examiner.

Establishing the Circumstances Leading to her Attendance

It is late in the evening so there must be something fairly significant to bring a new mother back to the maternity unit rather than trying to settle her baby down for the night.

Consider how you would establish a rapport with the patient and find out why she has come back to hospital so urgently that it could not wait until the next day. You should therefore assume she is likely to be distressed or upset and you should reflect on how to use a sympathetic approach to engage with her concerns as quickly as possible.

- Adequate information to be gathered from the patient:
  - Details related to her previous obstetric history
  - Details related to the series of events occurring from the time of her delivery (present pregnancy) until discharge
  - Check details of her labour, mode of delivery, postnatal course, and breastfeeding.
- Obtain details related to her present clinical condition.
- Ask specifically about presence of symptoms indicative of infection such as abdominal or perineal pain, bleeding, and discharge.

Marking Scheme

0	1	2	3	4	5	6
Fail		Borderline		Pass		

Counselling of the Patient

- Adopt an empathetic approach and appear to be dealing with the patient's concerns in a serious manner.
- Recognise the seriousness of a retained swab.
- Engage with the patient and do not try to sweep issues under the carpet.
- Demonstrate a good body language; maintain an excellent eye contact with the patient; lean forward while talking to the patient; occasionally nod while listening to the patient; seem to be taking her concerns seriously; and have an apology forthcoming.
- Recognise the patient's distress and concerns and deal empathetically with her.
- Avoid the use of medical jargon.
- Give a clear description of risk management process and how the patient would be contacted for an interrogation and a formal apology.

Addressing her Concerns

'Was the person who stitched my cuts and tears in the vaginal and anal region competent enough to be doing this on her own?'
- Explaining that all the SpRs are competent and assessed on their competencies before undertaking these procedures alone.
- A pre-selected labour ward consultant is always present on duty.

- Generally, the senior help is sought by the SpR or the coordinating midwife if some technical difficulties are encountered.
- Apologise to the role-player that the SpR involved is not available.

'How do you explain that the swab count appeared correct but one was left in my vagina?'

- Explain the process of checking the swab count at the end of the surgery.
- Admit that the swab was left inside.
- Swab count appeared correct at the end of the procedure.
- Acknowledge a mistake has been made and a full investigation will take place. An incident form has been filled and the matter would be evaluated at a higher level.
- Explain that her baby was big and there may have been an extension of the episiotomy cut until the anus (passage for faeces) which caused the bleeding and made repair and haemostasis difficult.

'I plan to take this further and want to register a complaint and seek legal advice. Whom do I contact?'

- The candidate should avoid being defensive and convey the role-player about the process of registering a complaint in a neutral manner. She should be advised to register her complaint first and then seek legal advice. She should be advised that once the legal team are involved, revelation of the investigations may be postponed.
- She should be advised to seek help from PALS (Patient Advice and Liaison Service). PALS serves as a point of contact for patients, their families, and their carers. It offers confidential advice, support and information about health-related matters, and the NHS complaints procedure.[6] Details of the nearest PALS can be obtained from the GP, or by calling NHS at 111.
- The patient can also complain to the commissioner of that service—either NHS England or the area Clinical Commissioning Group (CCG). While the most primary care services, such as GP and dental services, are commissioned by the NHS England, secondary care services, such as hospital care services, are commissioned by the CCG. The candidate can suggest providing the name and the address of chief executive.
- She should be advised that since the case triggered a risk management alert, a full investigation would have been begun in the hospital unit involved.

Marking Scheme

0	1	2	3	4	5	6
Fail		Borderline		Pass		

Patient Management

- Recognizes the need to take vaginal swabs and send them for histology.
- The competent candidate will also recognise the requirement to check the patient for further retained swabs and to take microbiology swabs.

- Explains that a retained swab is a 'never event' and confirms that shall report via Datix form (web-based incident reporting and risk management software).
- Should be able to demonstrate good understanding of adverse event reporting structures.
- Does not amplify the situation to the consultant on call or consultant he/she is booked under.
- The role-player should be advised regarding the immediate next steps to be taken.
- A course of appropriate antibiotics should be started.
- The competent candidate would also demonstrate good understanding of prescribing in patients who are breastfeeding.

Marking Scheme

0	1	2	3	4	5	6
Fail		Borderline		Pass		

Role-player's Score

The role-player can award a maximum of 2 marks to the candidate.

Marking Scheme

0	1	2
Role-player never wants to see candidate again	Role-player prepared to see candidate again	Role-player happy to see candidate again

Total score: /20

DISCUSSION

Issues

It is important for the candidate to recognise the requirement for apologising to this patient. There can be no excuse for leaving a swab in a patient after a procedure. A retained swab is therefore, described as a 'never event'.[7] All instruments, swabs and sharps, should be counted before and after every procedure. In case the count is not found to be correct, the procedure is not considered as complete until a search is made and the missing item found. This may include imaging the patent with the help of X-rays if required. It is important to apologise to the patient for the retained swab. This may seem as an unusual scenario because the candidate dealing with the role-player was actually not involved in the patient's care at all. However, in accordance with the principle of the 'duty of candour' all clinicians are obliged to acknowledge the occurrence of an untoward event and to express regret.[8] The duty of candour is the duty imposed on a public authority to assist the court in reaching the correct result, thereby improving the standard of health care. Instead, they must not seek to win the litigation at all costs.

Simultaneously, a review of the incident must be initiated by filling in an incident report, which must be eventually submitted to the clinical governance team. The apology provided to the patient does not imply that the candidate is admitting the guilt committed by their colleagues. This is just an essential aspect of being open and honest, an important component of clinical governance. There is good evidence that an early apology and acknowledgment of something going wrong by the health care professionals is likely to reduce the patient's anger, thereby decreasing the rate of litigation.

The candidate must take a good history in this case because in the examination there would be no title to guide the candidate. The candidate would have no idea about the retained swab until he/she starts talking to the role-player. This should give them a clue that they need to focus on their communication skills in order to deal with an upset or angry patient. The candidate should be able to display the skills for calming down the situation so that they can move on to the other parts of the task. Showing an empathic approach and offering a ready apology are likely to quickly calm down the role-player because she has been probably instructed to allow herself to be pacified so that the candidate can move on through other aspects of this station.

The next part of the station focuses on patient safety. The competent candidate should be able to demonstrate good understanding regarding the reporting structure for an adverse event and describe those processes to the simulated patient. The candidate should be able to explain the role-player that he/she would submit an electronic clinical incident form, the 'Datix' form, to ensure the automatic triggering off of the clinical governance processes on the next working day.

The third part of the station tests the candidate's ability to demonstrate their clinical knowledge. The candidate must demonstrate applied clinical knowledge by sending the swab to the histopathology department to confirm it is really a Raytec swab with a radio-opaque strip in it. The competent candidate will also identify the requirement for examining the patient to check for further retained swabs. They would also order microbiology swabs. Also, a competent candidate would start a course of appropriate antibiotics, simultaneously demonstrating that they have a good understanding of prescribing in patients who are breastfeeding.

Pitfalls

The major mistake, which candidates can commit on such type of station, is failing to recognising the seriousness of the event and trying to sweep the issues aside. Failing to apologise to the patient can also be considered as an important flaw.

Variations

Different variations which can be possible on such kind of stations could include a cases where there has been a medical error, for example leaving a swab, instrument or needle in the site of surgery or surgery which has not gone very well (for example, broken stitches, etc.)

OSCE STATION 5: ABNORMAL GLUCOSE TOLERANCE TEST

Candidate's Instructions

Mrs Noor Bano is a 28-year-old woman of Pakistani origin. She has visited your clinic at 22 weeks' of gestation for a detailed ultrasound scan of the baby.

The pregnancy appears to be progressing well. In view of her high risk for gestational diabetes, a 75-g glucose tolerance test (GTT) was performed, which revealed the following:

- Fasting blood sugar: 6.3 mmol/L
- 2 hours blood sugar: 9.6 mmol/L.

Her body mass index (BMI) was recorded as 28 kg/m^2, blood pressure (BP) 110/84 mmHg, haemoglobin 11.1 g%, mean corpuscular volume (MCV) 80 fL with normal electrophoresis. She had no other problems.

She is third gravida with one live child who is 6 years old. This baby was born by caesarean section in view of breech presentation. That baby weighed 2.8 kg at the time of birth. This surgery was performed in Pakistan. Though the surgery notes are not available with the patient, she tells you about the transverse scar on her abdomen. Five years ago she had a spontaneous miscarriage at 10 weeks of gestation.

This is a structured viva. The task is for 12 minutes (inclusive of 2 minutes of reading time). You have 10 minutes to answer the examiner's question. You shall be awarded marks for the following tasks:

Candidate's tasks:

- Critically evaluate the screening for diabetes mellitus in pregnancy
- Enumerate the risks of this pregnancy
- Describe your management at this stage in this patient?
- What postnatal advice would you give to this patient?

These tasks cover the domains as discussed next.

Core Clinical Skills Domains

Core clinical skills domains tested:

- Patient safety
- Information gathering
- Application of knowledge.

Module Tested

The module tested in station is Module 4 or 'Antenatal Care'.

EXAMINER'S INSTRUCTIONS AND STRUCTURED MARK SHEET

The examiner will mark the candidate on the basis of various tasks, which are allotted to the candidate. Out of a total score of 20, the examiner can award a maximum of 20 marks, which are distributed between various candidate tasks as shown next. Each candidate task would be globally scored by the examiner.

Screening for Diabetes Mellitus in Pregnancy

Screening for diabetes in pregnancy starts with a detailed obstetric and family history, which include the following:

- Previous history of macrosomic baby, unexplained stillbirth, congenital malformations (especially those common in diabetic pregnancies), polyhydramnios, etc.
- Family history of diabetes in a first-degree relative is associated with an increased risk of diabetes mellitus.
- Increased maternal weight is another risk factor.
- Race and age are also regarded as demographic risk factors.
- Identification of various risk factors such as glycosuria and recurrent infections, especially in the vulva and vagina, may indicate the requirement for screening.
- According to the ACHOIS (Australian Carbohydrate Intolerance Study in Pregnant Women) study, screening assumes an important role because treatment of cases of gestational diabetes is likely to reduce the risk of perinatal complications (Growther et al., 2005).[9] Most NHS trusts offer screening for gestational diabetes in form of a 2-hour 75-g oral GTT at 24–28 weeks of gestation to women with any one of the risk factors described above.

Marking Scheme

0	1	2	3	4	5	6
Fail		Borderline		Pass		

Risks of this Pregnancy

Maternal and foetal complications associated with gestational diabetes are tabulated in Table 8.3.

Marking Scheme

0	1	2	3	4
Fail		Borderline		Pass

Management

- Women with gestational diabetes mellitus should preferably be managed in a joint obstetric or diabetic clinic involving a multidisciplinary approach comprising of the obstetricians, diabetologists, dieticians, specialist nurses, midwives, etc.
- The patient is best treated with dietary and lifestyle changes alone. If the required blood glucose targets are not achieved through dietary changes and changes in lifestyle within 1–2 weeks, she should be prescribed metformin.[10,11] She can be prescribed insulin instead of metformin if metformin is contraindicated or unacceptable to the woman or if the blood

TABLE 8.3: Maternal and foetal complications related to gestational diabetes.

Maternal complications	Foetal/neonatal complications
Antepartum period: • Miscarriage • Pre-eclampsia • Preterm labour • Prolonged labour • Polyhydramnios (could be associated with foetal polyuria) • Shoulder dystocia • 35–50% risk of developing type II diabetes later in the life[17] • Increased risk of traumatic damage during labour • Increased risk of shoulder dystocia • Diabetic retinopathy and nephropathy can worsen rapidly during pregnancy • Difficulties assessing foetal growth and lie/presentation *Labour*: • Failure to progress • Shoulder dystocia • Trauma to the foetus—fractured clavicles, etc. • Difficult operative (abdominal and vaginal) deliveries • Venous thromboembolism	• Foetal distress and birth asphyxia • Brachial plexus injuries • Macrosomia or foetal birthweight more than 4 kg • Increased risk for perinatal death, birth trauma, and rates of caesarean section • Cephalohematoma, resulting in more pronounced neonatal jaundice • Stillbirth, congenital malformations, birth injury, and perinatal mortality • Hypoxia and sudden intrauterine death after 36 weeks' gestation • Congenital malformations • Foetal or neonatal hypoglycaemia, polycythaemia, hyperbilirubinaemia, and renal vein thrombosis • Hypomagnesaemia • Hypocalcaemia • Tetany • Neonatal jaundice • Polycythaemia • Stillbirths • An increased long-term risk of obesity and diabetes in the child

glucose targets are not being achieved with metformin.[11] Glibenclamide can be considered for women with gestational diabetes in whom blood glucose targets are not achieved with metformin, but who decline insulin therapy or who cannot tolerate metformin.[12] Plasma glucose levels must be maintained above 4 mmol/L in women on insulin or glibenclamide.

- *Foetal monitoring*: An individualised approach must be provided for monitoring foetal growth and well-being for women with diabetes. These include tests such as ultrasound monitoring of foetal growth and amniotic fluid volume every 4 weeks from 28 weeks to 36 weeks onwards.
- *Screening for congenital malformations*: First trimester ultrasound scan at 11–13 weeks must be done to measure nuchal translucency, as there is an increased risk of neural tube defects. Maternal serum screening for α-foetal proteins at 16–18 weeks must be done to rule out the risk for neural tube defects. Second trimester ultrasound scan for detailed scanning of foetal congenital anomalies must be performed at 18–20 weeks.[13] A detailed examination of the foetal heart (four chambers, outflow tracts, and three vessels) must also be performed at 20 weeks.
- Good glycaemic control must be achieved using regular blood glucose monitoring and HbA1c levels.
- *Renal assessment during pregnancy*: If renal assessment has not been undertaken in the preceding 3 months in women with pre-existing diabetes,

it should be done at the time of first antenatal visit during pregnancy. The patient may require a renal ultrasound depending on how the situation develops.

- The patient should be assessed at 36 weeks of gestation for deciding the mode of delivery in view of previous caesarean section.
- Aim must be to deliver the patient at 38–40 weeks' gestation depending on the diabetic control and baby's growth.
- Evaluation for maternal complications related to diabetes:
  - Urinary tract infections: MSU samples
  - Hypertension or pre-eclampsia: Checking blood pressure may be difficult, so larger cuffs must be used; regular checking of urine for proteinuria and nitrites
  - Diabetic complications: Hypoglycaemia, etc.

Marking Scheme

0	1	2	3	4	5	6
Fail		Borderline		Pass		

Postnatal Advice

- Immediately after birth, the insulin requirements may fall; therefore, insulin doses must be reduced immediately to prepregnancy levels, in order to avoid hypoglycaemia. Women with gestational diabetes whose blood glucose levels have returned to normal after the birth must be offered lifestyle advice (including weight control, diet, and exercise). Fasting plasma glucose levels must be tested 6–13 weeks after the birth to exclude diabetes.
- Breastfeeding improves insulin sensitivity and therefore is associated with reduced insulin requirements. As a result, adjustments of insulin dose are required.
- The woman must be counselled to lose weight before another pregnancy.
- Women with diabetes must be counselled regarding the importance of contraception and the requirement for preconception care when planning future pregnancies.
- Women who were diagnosed with gestational diabetes must be explained about the risks of gestational diabetes in future pregnancies, and be advised to get themselves tested for diabetes when planning future pregnancies.

Marking Scheme

0	1	2	3	4
Fail		Borderline		Pass

Total score: /20

DISCUSSION

Issues

Diabetes is one of the most common medical disorders of pregnancy, associated with a high perinatal morbidity and mortality. Although the risks associated with gestational diabetes are well recognised, it remains uncertain whether screening and treatment of gestational diabetes help to reduce the risk. NICE guidelines do not recommend screening. However, the recent ACHOIS study[9] has confirmed that screening and treatment significantly help in improving the outcome related to gestational diabetes. Screening is unable to identify all the cases of gestational diabetes because not all patients present with the pre-existing disease. Some patients are recognised for the first time in pregnancy, while some develop the disorder in pregnancy as a consequence of the diabetogenic effects of pregnancy.

Identification of at-risk groups is only the first step in the screening for diabetes mellitus. Following this, the definitive or second-stage screening must be offered, which is most commonly in the form of an oral GTT. In the UK and most of Europe, this is done with help of a 75-g glucose load (Table 8.4).[14,15] On the other hand, in the USA 100-g glucose load is used.

Pitfalls

This OSCE station is focusing on candidate's ability to apply clinical knowledge while confronted with a patient having gestational diabetes. Concentration on taking the history or highlighting the pointers to be elicited while taking the history can be considered as a potential mistake on such kind of stations. The candidate's answer must be precise and to the point. The candidate must exactly focus on the questions asked by the examiner.

Variations

Various variations in such kind of stations may include clinical scenarios where the candidate may be required to take a history from the role player (either with gestational diabetes or pre-existing diabetes) and counsel her regarding the various risks to her as well as her baby. Another scenario could involve a structured viva focusing on the patient with pre-existing diabetes.

TABLE 8.4: Diagnostic criteria for gestational diabetes mellitus for 75-g oral glucose tolerance test.

	WHO/NICE (mmol/L)	IADPSG* (mmol/L)
Fasting	≥5.6	≥5.1
1 hour	–	≥10.0
2 hour	≥7.8	≥8.5

(IADPSG: International Association of Diabetes and Pregnancy Study Groups; NICE: National Institute for Health and Care Excellence; WHO: World Health Organization)
Values for venous plasma samples.
*Diagnosis of gestational diabetes mellitus made if this value exceeded at any time point.

OSCE STATION 6: ANTEPARTUM HAEMORRHAGE

Candidate's Instructions

You are the duty obstetric registrar on the labour ward. You have been asked to see Jennifer Perkins, who has just been admitted with antepartum haemorrhage. She gives a history of falling on her abdomen last evening while she was playing with her child. Since then she has been having pain in the abdomen. She tried to sleep in the night. However, when she woke up in the morning, she was lying in a pool of blood and was very frightened. Her abdominal pain had also worsened. She was immediately brought to the hospital by an ambulance. It is estimated that she may have lost about 400–500 mL of blood.

Mrs Perkins is 32 years old in her second pregnancy and is presently 31 weeks pregnant. Her first child is 10 years old and was born via caesarean delivery. A transverse scar was given at the time of caesarean section. On admission the patient's BP was recorded at 120/70 mmHg with a pulse rate of 100 beats/min. She was alert and anxious. She was in extreme distress because she was having abdominal pain which appeared to be getting worse. She has also not felt any foetal movement since morning.

On abdominal examination, her uterus was tense and tender. It was difficult for you to locate the FHR using Doppler ultrasound scan. However, you ultimately managed to locate it on ultrasound and recorded a rate of approximately 110 beats/min. The patient was ultimately taken for an emergency caesarean delivery.

The task is for 12 minutes (inclusive of 2 minutes of reading time). This is a structured viva. You have 10 minutes to answer the examiner's questions. You shall be awarded marks for answering the examiner's following questions:

> **Candidate's tasks:**
> - What is the differential diagnosis in this case?
> - Outline your initial management of this patient.
> - What would be the future management plan in this patient?
> - What steps must be taken in the post-operative period?

These tasks cover the domains as discussed next.

Core Clinical Skills Domains

> **Core clinical skills domains tested:**
> - Patient safety
> - Information gathering
> - Application of knowledge.

Module Tested

The module tested in this station is Module 4 or 'Antenatal Care'.

EXAMINER'S INSTRUCTIONS AND STRUCTURED MARK SHEET

The examiner will mark the candidate on the basis of various tasks which are allotted to the candidate. Out of a total score of 20, the examiner can award a maximum of 20 marks, which are distributed between various candidate tasks as shown next. Each candidate task must be globally scored by the examiner.

The Likely Differential Diagnosis

The likely differential diagnosis in this case includes the following:
- Placental abruption (the clinical presentation in this case is pointing towards placental abruption; there is history of trauma and presence of uterine tenderness).
- Placenta praevia (unlikely in this case because the patient is experiencing severe abdominal and back pain; the bleeding in cases of placenta praevia is causeless and painless).
- Vasa praevia (unlikely in this case as there has been excessive bleeding and total foetal blood volume rarely exceeds 300 mL).
- Ruptured uterus (a transverse scar is unlikely to rupture in the antenatal period).
- Placental edge bleed.
- Presence of cervical tumour or other local causes (these causes can be excluded on per speculum examination).

Marking Scheme

0	1	2	3	4
Fail	Borderline		Pass	

Initial Management Plan

- A rapid assessment of the patient needs to be undertaken, so that she can be stabilized.
- Monitoring of vitals (pulse, blood pressure, etc.) at every 15–30 minute intervals depending upon the severity of bleeding.
- The candidate needs to assess whether the bleeding continuing, and if so they need to assess how much overall volume loss has occurred.
- Insertion of a central venous pressure (CVP) line, IV line, and a urinary catheter. IV access must be preferably established with a 14-gauge cannula.
- Administration of IV fluids (normal saline or Hartmann's) or Haemaccel® depending on the overall clinical picture.
- Blood to be sent for ABO and Rh typing, cross-matching (usually 4–6 units depending on the assessment) and CBC, including coagulation profile, urea and electrolytes, and liver function tests.
- Blood transfusion must be started if signs of shock are present.
- The foetal heart sounds must be monitored continuously.
- Abdomen must be palpated for tenderness.

- Review the notes to see if there are any underlying problems with the pregnancy.
- Since this appears to be a clear cut case of placental abruption, the doctor on duty must inform the labour ward consultant, anaesthetist, and the haematologist. In case of doubt, the placental position must be localised using an ultrasound scan. When the delivery is approaching, the paediatrician also needs to be called.

Marking Scheme

0	1	2	3	4	5	6
Fail		Borderline		Pass		

Future Management

- Diagnosis in this case most likely appears to be placental abruption.
- Once the patient has been stabilized and her bloods are taken, further management depends on the clinical picture and the presence or absence of the foetal heart.
- Definitive treatment in these cases is the delivery of the baby. In case of severe abruption, delivery should be performed by the fastest possible route. Caesarean delivery needs to be performed for most cases with severe placental abruption.
- If there are no concerns about the placental location or other local cervical causes, vaginal digital examination needs to be done to see whether the cervix is dilating and vaginal delivery would be possible.
- If the baseline bradycardia persists, a category I unplanned emergency caesarean section (Table 8.5) would be required to deliver the baby before the foetal heart is completely lost.[16]
- Intramuscular corticosteroids need to be administered to the mother in this case in lieu of foetal prematurity.
- Resuscitation must be continued on the way to theatre and the circulating volume needs to be restored.
- Consent form needs to be signed.
- The patient is at a risk of developing disseminated intravascular coagulation (DIC). Blood coagulation profile needs to be done at every 2 hourly intervals.

TABLE 8.5: NCEPOD classification system for caesarean delivery on the basis of urgency.[16]

Type	Category	Description
Unplanned CS	1	Immediate threat to the life of the woman or foetus
	2	Maternal or foetal compromise which is not immediately life-threatening
Planned CS	3	No maternal or foetal compromise, but nevertheless early delivery is required
	4	Delivery timed to suit woman or staff

(NCEPOD: National Confidential Enquiry into Patient Outcome and Death; CS: caesarean section)

If she develops a coagulopathy then liaison with the haematologist is required for correcting this.

- Documentation of the input and output of fluids needs to be maintained.
- Catheterisation may be done and an hourly record of urine volume be maintained.
- Insertion of CVP line may be required depending on the clinical situation.
- As a rule of thumb, for every 6 units of red cells transfused, 4 units of fresh frozen plasma (FFP) must be administered.[17]
- Transfusion of platelet concentrate may be required if the platelet count is less than 50×10^9/L.
- Transfusion of cryoprecipitate may be required if fibrinogen levels are less than 1.0 g/dL
- Intramuscular corticosteroids need to be administered to the mother in this case in lieu of foetal prematurity.

Marking Scheme

0	1	2	3	4	5	6
Fail		Borderline		Pass		

Post-operative Management

- Risk management form needs to be filled as there has been massive bleeding.
- Consider the admission of the patient in high-dependency unit. However, joint decision in collaboration with the anaesthetist needs to be made.
- Vital signs need to be continuously monitored.
- Amount of blood loss also needs to be monitored.
- Intravenous syntocinon infusion must be continued over the next 6–12 hours based on the patient's clinical picture and the amount of bleeding.
- Urine input and output must be monitored on an hourly basis.
- Thromboprophylaxis in form of anti-embolism stockings (with or without) heparin infusion and early mobilisation.

Marking Scheme

0	1	2	3	4
Fail	Borderline		Pass	

Total score: /20

DISCUSSION

Issues

In cases of antepartum haemorrhage, it is important for the candidate to apply their clinical knowledge in order to differentiate between the various causes of antepartum haemorrhage such as placenta praevia, placental abruption, etc.

Pitfalls

One of the major mistakes, which a candidate can commit in such types of station is a failure to differentiate between the various causes of antepartum haemorrhage.

Variations

Variations in this kind of station could include scenarios representing various causes of antepartum haemorrhage (e.g. placenta praevia, placental abruption, etc.). The scenario could also be associated with one of the complications of antepartum haemorrhage (e.g. requirement for blood transfusion in Jehovah's witnesses or DIC in association with placental abruption).

OSCE STATION 7: ASTHMA IN PREGNANCY

Candidate's Instructions

You are an ST5 working in the clinic. You are about to see Mrs Lisa Macdonald, a 35-year-old woman, who has been referred by her GP. The referral letter from the GP is as follows:

Windy Ridge Surgery Cliff Top Road Strathclyde ST5 5BB
Dear Obstetrician,
Re: Lisa McDonald, 35 years old
Please could you see Ms Lisa McDonald who was diagnosed with asthma at the age of 10 years. For the last 15 years, she has been experiencing acute severe asthmatic attacks. On an average, she gets hospitalized at least once in a year. She has a 4-year-old daughter who was delivered at 32 weeks of gestation by caesarean section because Mrs McDonald had experienced a significant deterioration of her respiratory function. The baby was born preterm and was small for dates. The baby was admitted in the special care baby unit for about 3 months before being handed over to her parents.

Mrs Macdonald smokes about 5–10 cigarettes a day. Her BMI is 31 kg/m^2 and she is trying to lose weight. She has a new partner and wants to have a baby with him. However, she is concerned about the risks to herself as well as her baby in lieu of her asthma, her asthmatic medications, and previous caesarean delivery. She would like to receive more information regarding the possible implications of her pregnancy on her baby as well as herself. The medication, which she is currently taking for her asthma, includes the following: prednisolone 40 mg daily, budesonide (Pulmicort® CFC-free inhaler, 100 μg); ipratropium bromide (Atrovent®) nebulisers; montelukast (Singulair®) tablets, 10 mg daily; and Pulvinal® salbutamol inhaler (200 μg).

Yours sincerely,
Dr Louis Andrews (FRCGP)

The task is for 12 minutes (inclusive of 2 minutes of reading time). You have 10 minutes to counsel her about the situation. You shall be awarded marks for the following tasks:

Candidate's tasks:

- Take the relevant history from the patient
- Outline a specific management plan for the patient before and during pregnancy
- Address the patient's concerns.

These tasks cover the domains as discussed next.

Core Clinical Skills Domains

Core clinical skills domains tested:

- Patient safety
- Communication with patients
- Communication with colleagues
- Information gathering
- Application of knowledge.

Module Tested

The module tested in this station is Module 5 or 'Maternal Medicine'.

Role-player's Brief

You are Lisa McDonald, a 35-year-old woman, working as a part-time secretary in a lawyer's office. You were first diagnosed with asthma at the age of 10 years. Initially the condition was reasonably mild and stable and you had been prescribed an inhaler by your GP. However, since last few years your asthmatic attacks have severely deteriorated and have become more severe and frequent. You have been hospitalized several times since past 5–6 years due to sudden severe asthmatic attacks and you have been now prescribed both inhalers and tablets to help with your breathing.

You have been married since past 10 years. You have one girl child, Ann from this marriage who is 4 years old. While you were pregnant with Ann, your asthma had really deteriorated and you were admitted in the hospital right from about 26 weeks of pregnancy. By the time you reached 32 weeks of gestation, your breathlessness had really deteriorated. As a result, you were delivered at 32 weeks by caesarean section. After delivery, you were shifted to the intensive care unit because of concerns about your asthma and breathing. Your daughter was born preterm and weighed less than 3 pounds. She was admitted in the special care baby unit for about 3 months. It took you almost 6 months to normalise after delivery.

You smoke 5–10 cigarettes each day. Your GP has advised you several times to give up smoking. Your GP had also referred you to a stop-smoking service and advised you to try nicotine replacement. However, you never took help of these services because you had decided that you would never want to become pregnant again.

You have now divorced your previous husband. You have a new partner and you would like to have a baby with him. However, you are worried about the risks, which you or your baby may face. You would like to know all the possible information regarding the complications to you and your baby because of your asthma, the medications you are taking as well as your previous caesarean section. You feel that the medications that you are presently taking appear to be working well and able to keep your asthma under reasonable control.

Prompt Questions

- Will my asthma worsen again during my pregnancy?
- Could I die during my delivery?

- Can my asthma or the medications I am taking for asthma cause harm to my baby?
- Will I need another caesarean section?

EXAMINER'S INSTRUCTIONS AND STRUCTURED MARK SHEET

The examiner will mark the candidate on the basis of various tasks which are allotted to the candidate. Out of a total score of 20, the examiner can award a maximum of 18 marks, which are distributed between various candidate tasks as shown next. The role-player can award a maximum of 2 marks to the candidate. Each candidate task must be globally scored by the examiner.

Taking Relevant History

- Gather information regarding the present condition of the woman's asthma.
- Series of events related to asthma which occurred during her first pregnancy both in terms of her antenatal admission and her post-operative recovery need to be defined.
- The candidate needs to enquire from the role-player her present condition in comparison to her condition before her first pregnancy.
- History related to asthmatic medications, she is currently undertaking.
- Previous obstetric history in details.
- The competent candidate will enquire about the role-player's smoking habits and also emphasise the requirement to provide support to help her quit smoking. Quitting smoking is not only likely to help improve her asthma, it is also likely to help maximise her chances for a successful pregnancy.

Marking Scheme

0	1	2	3	4	5	6
Fail		Borderline		Pass		

Management Plan for the Patient

- The candidate needs to offer a possible management plan wherein they must optimise asthma control before conception.
- A reliable method of contraception must be used until Mrs McDonald's condition has been optimised.
- Referral to smoking cessation services.
- Advise the role-player to meet her GP for nicotine replacement therapy.

Care during Pregnancy

- Offering reassurance to the patient that once she is pregnant, she would have access to multidisciplinary care that would promptly treat any asthma attack.
- The most appropriate method of delivery would also be decided by the multidisciplinary team depending upon the patient's clinical situation.

- The situation could be life-threatening if untreated or poorly managed. The competent candidate would communicate the risks to both the mother and the baby in an empathetic manner without scaring the patient.
- The competent candidate would encourage the patient to make an informed choice regarding the risks involved and whether or not she wants to have another baby.
- The risks to the mother not only relate to the asthmatic condition, but other treatment-related risks to the women, e.g. risk of thrombosis due to prolonged hospitalisation and the risk of gestational diabetes as a result of steroid administration. If the mother's asthmatic condition further worsens, vaginal birth after caesarean (VBAC) may not be possible and the woman may require a repeat caesarean delivery. There is a significant risk for the foetus to be prematurely born.
- *Risks related to the use of various asthma-related drugs:*[18] The role-player should be reassured regarding the use of prednisolone, which does not cause foetal abnormalities. She should be reassured that salbutamol inhaler can be taken as usual during pregnancy. Though salbutamol may be secreted in small amounts into the breast milk, salbutamol inhalers can be used as usual by the breastfeeding women, because negligible amount of medicine passes into the breast milk after using an inhaler. This is unlikely to harm the baby. Presently there is limited safety data available related to the use of montelukast. Therefore, the candidate would need to consult the local drug information service. As a result, montelukast should be prescribed in pregnancy only if its benefits clearly exceed its risks. The candidate may need to consult the local drug information service before prescribing this drug.
- *Advice related to smoking*: If she is still smoking, smoking cessation forms an important part of management especially in this case to reduce the symptoms of asthma and improve the efficacy of inhaled corticosteroids.[19]

Marking Scheme

0	1	2	3	4	5	6
Fail		Borderline		Pass		

Addressing the Patient's Concerns

- Various probable complications to the mother and baby due to asthma, repeat caesarean delivery, and complications related to the asthmatic drugs must be explained to the patient. The role-player must be counselled about significant risk of deterioration in the asthmatic condition during her pregnancy, which could be life-threatening. Risks involved to the baby include increased perinatal mortality or morbidity due to premature delivery. Other risks to the foetus include growth restriction and adrenal suppression due to high-dose steroids. Both these risks must also be clearly explained to the patient.

- Without scaring the patient, a competent candidate must be able to explain the role-player that under extreme circumstances it may even be necessary to make decisions regarding whether to save life of the mother or the baby.
- Patient needs to be counselled that risk related to the use of asthmatic medicines is less than that associated with that related to uncontrolled asthma during pregnancy.
- Provide advice related to the potential risks or complications of another pregnancy.
- Risk due to asthma can be considerably reduced if the patient asthma is well controlled prior to pregnancy.
- Negotiate a plan with the patient whether she wants to become pregnant or avoid pregnancy based on the various complications explained to her.

Marking Scheme

0	1	2	3	4	5	6
Fail		Borderline		Pass		

Role-player's Score

The role-player can award a maximum of 2 marks to the candidate.

Marking Scheme

0	1	2
Role-player never wants to see candidate again	Role-player prepared to see candidate again	Role-player happy to see candidate again

Total score: /20

DISCUSSION

Issues

This is a preconception counselling session and tests the candidate's counselling skills based on his/her clinical knowledge. The candidate must discuss potentially life-threatening asthmas without unduly scaring the patient. The candidate has to negotiate with the simulated patient in a way as to help her reach a shared-decision. The patient could choose to become pregnant or avoid pregnancy based on the candidate's advice. The candidate must consider safety of the patient as well as her baby while prescribing her asthmatic drugs. Multidisciplinary approach of management must also be explained to the role-player. The candidate must not use medical terminology while explaining the risks to the patient. The candidate must counsel the patient on the basis of her experience with her first pregnancy and her consequent progress. Using this approach, the candidate must demonstrate the probable risks to the role-player.

Pitfalls

Good counselling skills are especially important in this type of station. Frightening the patient or forcing her to make a clinical decision is an important mistake which the candidate must not commit. The candidate should make use of his/her negotiation skills to enable the role-player make a decision using shared decision-making. Not directing the role-player towards a shared decision making and forcing her to make a particular decision can be considered as a potential pitfall for this kind of station.

Variations

The variations in this kind of stations could include discussion pertaining to any other medical illness co-existing with pregnancy, e.g. underlying heart disease, chronic hypertension, diabetes mellitus (type 1 and 2), etc.

OSCE STATION 8: INFERTILITY DUE TO POLYCYSTIC OVARIAN DISEASE

Candidate's Instructions

Mrs Carolyn Devine is a 33-year-old woman with primary infertility since past 2 years, who is experiencing irregular bleeding since past 6 months. She has been referred to your outpatient clinic by her GP. She was originally seen in the clinic 3 months ago and some baseline investigations were undertaken. Results of these investigations are described below.

The Surgery Blackhorse Road
London E44
Dear Doctor,
Re: Mrs Carolyn Devine, 33 years old patient
Can you please see Mrs Carolyn Devine who has a history of primary infertility over past 2 years. Presently, Mrs Carolyn is 33 years old with a history of irregular periods over past 6 months. She was diagnosed as a case of endometriosis on laparoscopy 1 year ago. On laparoscopic examination, the endometriotic spots were found on the uterosacral ligaments. The rest of the pelvis appeared normal. Carolyn had been on a course of Provera for 9 months following laparoscopy and is now asymptomatic.

General physical examination is unremarkable with a BP of 110/70 mmHg and a BMI = 32. Pelvic examination is normal.

Yours sincerely,
Mr A Sherman (MRCGP)

Investigations: Semen analysis for Derick Devine, partner of Carolyn Devine
- Collection: Masturbation
- Days abstinence: 1 day
- Time since production: 90 minutes
- Volume: 2.8 mL
- Viscosity: <3

- Normal motility: 50%
- Sperm concentration: 25 million/mL
- Abnormal form: 30%
- Non-sperm cell concentration: 0.3 million/mL
- Total motile sperm: >50%
- Tray agglutination test: No antisperm antibody detected

Investigations (Carolyn Devine)
- *Serum testosterone levels*: 4.2 nmol/L (normal value 0.5–1.8 nmol/L)
- *Luteinising hormone (LH) levels*: 42 IU/L (normal value 2–10 IU/L)
- *Follicle-stimulating hormone (FSH) levels*: 6 IU/L (normal value 2–8 IU/L)
- *Hysterosalpingogram (HSG)*: The uterus is normal, anteverted, and mobile. Bilateral uterine tubes fill up uniformly with dye. The isthmus and ampullary portions of both the tubes appear normal. A bilateral free spill of contrast occurs into the peritoneal cavity with little dye retention.
- *Pelvic ultrasound*: Ultrasound shows normal anteverted uterus, with an enlarged right ovary and normal looking left ovary. Right ovary shows multiple small follicles in the periphery. No other pelvic pathology is observed. No fluid is observed in the pouch of Douglas.
- *High vaginal swab (HVS) result*: Normal commensals; endocervical swab: negative for chlamydia.

The task is for 12 minutes (inclusive of 2 minutes of reading time). You have 10 minutes to carry out the following tasks:

Candidate's tasks:

- Discuss an appropriate supplementary history
- Discuss the results of investigations
- What are the important aspects of polycystic ovary syndrome (PCOS) that you need to discuss with the woman?
- Discuss appropriate management options.

These tasks cover the domains as discussed next.

Core Clinical Skills Domains

Core clinical skills domains tested:

- Patient safety
- Communication with patients
- Communication with colleagues
- Information gathering
- Application of knowledge.

Module Tested

The module tested in this station is Module 10 or 'Subfertility'.

Role-player's Brief

- You are Carolyn Devine, a 33-year-old woman, who works as a sales assistant in the super market.
- You commenced your periods at the age of 11 years and had been having a regular 28-day cycle with bleeding for 5 days. You experienced mild discomfort during your periods which subsided on taking pain killers.

- You have been married to Derick Devine, your husband, for past 8 years. Initially you used oral contraceptive pills during the first 5 years of your marriage. Now you have been trying to conceive since past 2 years and have regular intercourse, three times a week. You have been experiencing irregular periods since past 6 months. Your periods have lately become extremely infrequent and since past 6 months, you had only 2 periods. Amount of bleeding has also become scanty and your periods have now lasted for 3–4 days.
- You have not experienced any symptoms such as excessive growth of facial hair, acne, deepening of voice, etc.
- One year ago you underwent a laparoscopy as an investigation for pain during intercourse. You were diagnosed as a case of mild endometriosis and were successfully treated with diathermy at the time of surgery. You had been on a course of Provera for 9 months following laparoscopy. Rest of your past gynaecological history is non-significant.
- Your past medical and surgical history is also unremarkable and you are not taking any medication.
- Your last smear was prior to your referral and the result was normal.
- You are a non-smoker and non-alcoholic. You have not used any recreational drug in the past.
- Your husband is otherwise fit and well and works at a vehicle repair shop. He on an average smokes 5–10 cigarettes per day and occasionally drinks a glass of wine with meals. He has never fathered a child in the past.
- You are getting worried and disheartened because you and your husband are presently longing to become parents. You have further become tensed up because of your advancing age. You have heard that a woman's fertility significantly decreases after the age of 35 years.
- The results of the various investigations would suggest the underlying factor to be polycystic ovarian disease. The candidate should be able to explain the various management options available to you.

Prompt Questions

- Will I be ever able to become a mother in future?
- What treatment options are available to me?
- How can this problem affect my future health?

EXAMINER'S INSTRUCTIONS AND STRUCTURED MARK SHEET

The examiner will mark the candidate on the basis of various tasks which are allotted to the candidate. Out of a total score of 20, the examiner can award a maximum of 18 marks, which are distributed between various candidate tasks as shown next. The role-player can award a maximum of 2 marks to the candidate. Each candidate task must be globally scored by the examiner.

History

Relevant history, which needs to be elicited:
- History of infrequent periods (oligomenorrhoea):
    - Frequency of periods
    - Their duration
    - History of pain during periods.
- *Features suggestive of hyperandrogenism*: Increased growth of facial hair (hirsutism), acne, etc.
- Obstetric and gynaecologal history
- Past medical or surgical history
- Check about coital frequency
- Ask about LMP (it is important to check the LMP in this case because she may already be pregnant).

Marking Scheme

0	1	2	3	4
Fail		Borderline		Pass

Discussion of the Results of Investigations

- Results of various investigations which must be performed in the suspected cases of PCOS are enlisted in Table 8.6.[20]
- Diagnosis of PCOS is made after exclusion of differential diagnosis such as thyroid dysfunction, congenital adrenal hyperplasia, hyperprolactinaemia, adrenal tumours, and Cushing's syndrome. In suspected cases thyroid function tests or serum prolactin levels must be performed accordingly.
- Rotterdam criteria for diagnosis of PCOS are described in the Box 8.1. Diagnosis of PCOS should be made, when two of the three criteria as described in Box 8.1 are met.[21]

TABLE 8.6: Serum parameters which are altered in cases of PCOD.

Normal levels	Levels in PCOD
Serum testosterone (0.5–1.8 nmol/L)	Increased levels of androgens (testosterone and androstenedione)
SHBG (16–119 nmol/L)	Reduced levels of SHBG
Free androgen index (testosterone levels × 100/SHBG) <5	Increased free androgen index
FSH (2–8 IU/L)	Reduced/normal FSH levels
LH (2–10 IU/L)	Increased LH levels
Anti-Müllerian hormone (35 pmol/L)	Increased
Serum oestradiol/oestrogen levels	Increased
Fasting insulin levels (<30 mU/L)	Increased

(PCOD: polycystic ovary disease; SHBG: sex hormone-binding globulins; FSH: follicle-stimulating hormone; LH: luteinising hormone)

> **BOX 8.1:** Rotterdam criteria for diagnosis of polycystic ovary syndrome.
>
> 1. Infrequent or absent ovulation (anovulation)
> 2. Clinical or biochemical features of hyperandrogenism, such as excessive hair growth, acne, raised luteinising hormone, and raised androgen levels
> 3. Polycystic ovaries: Morphologically, there is bilateral enlargement, thickened ovarian capsule, multiple follicular cysts (usually ranging between 2 mm to 8 mm in diameter), and an increased amount of stroma.
>
> Features of polycystic ovarian morphology on ultrasound scan are as follows (Fig. 8.2):[20]
> • Greater than 12 follicles measuring between 2 mm to 9 mm in diameter, located peripherally, resulting in a pearl necklace appearance.
> • Increased echogenicity of ovarian stroma and/or ovarian volume >10 mL. The distribution of the follicles is not required, with one ovary being sufficient for the diagnosis.

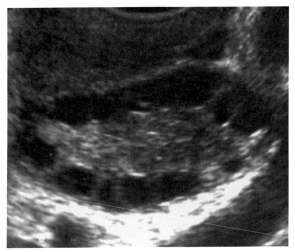

Fig. 8.2: Ultrasound features of polycystic ovarian morphology.

Marking Scheme

0	1	2	3	4	5
Fail		Borderline		Pass	

Important Aspects of PCOS

Important aspects of PCOS, which need to be discussed with the woman, are:
- *Type 2 diabetes mellitus*: She should be informed about the risk of developing insulin resistance, resulting in impaired glucose tolerance and type 2 diabetes mellitus.
- *Ischaemic heart disease*: She should also be communicated about the long-term risks of developing cardiovascular disease, especially ischaemic heart disease due to abnormal cholesterol metabolism in the future.
- *Sleep apnoea*: If the woman's BMI raised, she is at an increased risk of developing sleep apnoea.

- *Endometrial cancer*: Due to unopposed action of oestrogens on the uterine endometrium, the woman is also at an increased risk of endometrial hyperplasia and carcinoma. Regular withdrawal bleeds are recommended in order to prevent this.
- *Breast cancer*: There is inconclusive evidence regarding the association of PCOS with breast cancer. However, factors such as obesity, hyper-androgenism, and infertility, which may be associated with PCOS, also act as the risk factors for breast cancer. A recent meta-analysis, however, has demonstrated that PCOS does not increase the risk of the breast cancer.[22] Further prospective cohort studies are needed to provide convincing evidence to show whether or not PCOS can increase the risk of the breast cancer. Therefore, watchful vigilance is required in the form of regular breast examination and mammography amongst such patients.
- *Ovarian cancer*: This is more likely to be related to the ovulation-inducing drugs rather than PCOS per se. Therefore, patients with PCOS undergoing infertility treatment with ovulation inducing drugs must be followed up with a high index of suspicion since symptoms of ovarian cancer are usually vague and non-specific.

Implications of PCOS in Relation to Pregnancy

Since the patient keenly desires pregnancy in this case, the implications which PCOS can have on her pregnancy need to be explained to her:
- Medical or surgical assistance for induction of ovulation would be required in most of the cases.
- Although the ovulation rate with most of the regimens is high in cases of PCOS, pregnancy rates are much lower. There is an increased risk of miscarriage. Moreover, these agents are associated with an increased risk of multiple pregnancies as well as ovarian hyperstimulation syndrome.
- The patient needs to be aware about the early symptoms of diabetes mellitus and have regular check-ups with the GP.
- Screening for gestational diabetes less than 20 weeks' gestation and managed accordingly.
- Other problems related to raised BMI need to be explained to her (e.g. hypertension/operative delivery).

Marking Scheme

0	1	2	3	4
Fail		Borderline		Pass

Discussion of Appropriate Treatment Options

- *Lifestyle changes*: Lifestyle changes for reducing her weight are likely to help in significantly improving her fertility.
  - *General health advice*: Adequate and regular exercise
  - *Dietary advice*: For reducing the cholesterol levels
  - Early warning signs of heart disease or attacks need to be kept in mind

- *Hypertension*: These patients may be at an increased risk of developing hypertension in future. Therefore, their blood pressure needs to be regularly checked. Complaints of persistent headaches need to be immediately looked into because this may be associated with severe underlying hypertension.
- *Cardiovascular disease*: Early warning signs of heart disease or attacks need to be kept in mind.
- *Insulin-sensitizing agents*: Insulin-sensitizing agents (e.g. metformin) may be useful in improving insulin resistance.
- Weight-reduction drugs may be helpful in reducing insulin resistance.
- *Strategies for improving her fertility*: Lifestyle changes for reducing her weight, drugs for inducing ovulation, and laparoscopic drilling of the ovaries, will significantly help in improve her fertility.

Role of Surgery in Patients with PCOS

- Ovarian drilling should be reserved for selected infertile women with an ordinary BMI.
- Bariatric surgery may be a possible option depending on local protocols.

Marking Scheme

0	1	2	3	4	5
Fail		Borderline		Pass	

Role-player's Score

The role-player can award a maximum of 2 marks to the candidate.

Marking Scheme

0	1	2
Role-player never wants to see candidate again	Role-player prepared to see candidate again	Role-player happy to see candidate again

Total score: /20

DISCUSSION

Issues

The station assesses the candidate's ability to interpret the clinical findings and the results of various investigations. The candidate must have some idea regarding the normal values for various investigations; especially those related to infertility so that they can quickly interpret the results in the examination. It is unlikely that there will be a role-play couple in the examination; usually there may be a woman or sometimes her partner. The candidate must focus both on the male and female factors related to infertility. Though the diagnosis is obvious in the stations related to infertility, it is always important for the candidate to critically appraise the various treatment options which would be feasible for the couple. They also need to assess how far the couple is prepared to travel along the road of assisted reproductive technologies.

The diagnosis in this case is PCOS. Therefore, the patient is at an increased risk of cardiovascular disorders, including hypertension and ischaemic heart disease. The patient must be advised to look out for early warning signs of hypertension and ischaemic heart disease, such as headaches, easy fatigability, shortness of breath, and precordial chest pain. She must visit her GP regularly, who needs to monitor the patient's blood pressure and cholesterol levels and examine her cardiovascular system regularly.

Since she is also at an increased risk of developing insulin resistance, she must therefore be educated on the early symptoms of diabetes mellitus, such as polyuria, polydipsia, and polyphagia. She must also visit her GP clinic regularly for urine testing and estimation of blood-glucose levels.

Another important complication of PCOS is the development of endometrial cancer. In cases of PCOS, endometrial cancer may occur before menopause. Irregular bleeding is a recognised symptom of PCOS and may also be a presentation for endometrial cancer; therefore, the patient may consult her GP if she experiences any unusual vaginal bleeding. She should be prescribed cyclical progestogens to counteract the unopposed action of oestrogens over the uterine endometrium. Ultrasound scan, endometrial biopsy, and hysteroscopic assessment of the endometrium may be required to rule out endometrial cancer.

Appropriate dietary and exercise advice is especially important in this case as the patient has increased BMI. However, advice related to dietary changes and exercise must be offered whether or not she is obese. Weight loss will not only help in reducing the risk of the health issues, such as hypertension and endometrial cancer, but will also reduce the risks of diabetes and insulin resistance.

Pitfalls

Concentrating just on taking a history can be considered as an important pitfall in these types of stations. Although history taking is important, the candidates need to divide their time in four candidate tasks: history taking; discussion regarding the results of investigations; discussion regarding the important health aspects of PCOS; and critical appraisal of the management. The candidate must not simply outline or discuss the management.

Variations

Different kinds of variations which are possible for such kind of stations are diverse scenarios, where the results of the investigations point towards different other causes of infertility (e.g. male factor infertility, endometriosis, tubal factor infertility, etc.).

REFERENCES

1. Waitzkin H. Doctor-patient communication. Clinical implications of social scientific research. JAMA. 1984;252(17):2441-6.

2. National Institute of Clinical Excellence. (2015). Preterm labour and birth. NICE guideline [NG25]. London: NICE.
3. American College of Obstetricians and gynaecologists. (2017). Antenatal Corticosteroid Therapy for Fetal Maturation. Committee opinion No. 713. [online] Available from www.acog.org/Resources-And-Publications/Committee-Opinions/Committee-on-Obstetric-Practice/Antenatal-Corticosteroid-Therapy-for-Fetal-Maturation. [Accessed October 2017].
4. Creasy RK, Gummer BA, Liggins GC. System for predicting spontaneous preterm birth. Obstet Gynecol. 1980;55(6):692-5.
5. National Institute of Clinical Excellence. (updated 2017) Intrapartum care for healthy women and babies (CG190). NICE: London.
6. Improving Independent Complaints Advocacy in Health and Social Care: Background and Position Briefing. Healthwatch England. November 2013.
7. Coates T. Retained swabs? A never event that has the potential to act as a fundamental driver to improve practice and systems. J Perioper Pract. 2012;22(4):112-3.
8. Jacob H, Raine J. Openness and honesty when things go wrong: the professional duty of candour (GMC guideline). Arch Dis Child Educ Pract Ed. 2016;101(5):243-5.
9. Growther CA, Hiller JE, Moss JR, et al. Effect of gestational diabetes mellitus on pregnancy outcomes (the Achois Trial). NEJM. 2005;352:2477-86.
10. Landon MB, Spong CY, Thom E, et al. A multicenter, randomized trial of treatment for mild gestational diabetes. N Engl J Med. 2009;361(14):1339-48.
11. Rowan JA, Hague WM, Gao W, et al; MiG Trial Investigators. Metformin versus insulin for the treatment of gestational diabetes. N Engl J Med. 2008;358(19):2003-15.
12. Langer O, Conway DL, Berkus MD, et al. A comparison of glyburide and insulin in women with gestational diabetes mellitus. N Engl J Med. 2000;343(16):1134-8.
13. Miller E, Hare JW, Cloherty JP, et al. Elevated maternal hemoglobin A1c in early pregnancy and major congenital anomalies in infants of diabetic mothers. N Engl J Med. 1981;304(22):1331-4.
14. Metzger BE, Gabbe SG, Persson B, et al. International association of diabetes and pregnancy study group's recommendations on the diagnosis and classification of hyperglycemia in pregnancy. Diabetes Care. 2010;33(3):676-82.
15. National Institute for Health and Clinical Excellence. NICE clinical guideline 63: Diabetes in pregnancy: Management from preconception to the postnatal period. London: NICE; 2015. [online] Available from https://www.nice.org.uk/guidance/ng3. [Accessed October 2017].
16. National Confidential Enquiry into Perioperative Deaths (NCEPOD). (1995). Report of the National Confidential Enquiry into Perioperative Deaths 1992/3. [online] Available from www.ncepod.org.uk/1992report. [Accessed October 2017].
17. Royal College of Obstetricians and gynaecologists. Antepartum Haemorrhage. Green-top Guideline No. 63; November 2011.
18. Lim A, Hussainy SY, Abramson MJ. Asthma drugs in pregnancy and lactation. Aust Prescr. 2013;36:5-61.
19. Goldie MH, Brightling CE. Asthma in pregnancy. The Obstetrician & Gynaecologist. 2013;15:241-5.
20. Michelmore KF, Balen AH, Dunger DB, et al. Polycystic ovaries and associated clinical and biochemical features in young women. Clin Endocrinol (Oxf). 1999;51(6):779-86.
21. Rotterdam ESHRE/ASRM-Sponsored PCOS consensus workshop group. Revised 2003 consensus on diagnostic criteria and long-term health risks related to polycystic ovary syndrome (PCOS). Hum Reprod. 2004;19(1):41-7.
22. Shobeiri F, Jenabi E. The association between polycystic ovary syndrome and breast cancer: a meta-analysis. Obstet Gynecol Sci. 2016;59(5):367-72.

9

Ethics, Medico-Legal Issues, and Clinical Governance

CLINICAL GOVERNANCE

A systematic approach by NHS for sustaining and improving the quality of patient care is described as clinical governance.[1]

Clinical governance has been defined by the Department of Health as '*A framework through which NHS organisations are accountable for continually improving the quality of their services and safeguarding high standards of care by creating an environment in which excellence in clinical care will flourish.*'[2]

The concept of clinical governance is mainly determined by four words in this definition: framework, accountability, quality of services, and environment.

- *Framework*: This is the structure/skeleton which provides a basis for delivering high-quality healthcare services, thereby enabling all the healthcare professionals to follow a set pattern.
- *Accountability*: This is a concept of clinical governance through which every individual working in any NHS organisation is answerable for the quality of his/her work to their senior healthcare professionals within the organisation. These could include the head of the department, chief executive officer or medical/clinical director.
- *Quality for services*: The clinicians must maintain high quality of services by following evidence-based practice, and evaluating and optimising the process of care.
- *Environment for implementation*: All NHS organisations must have systems in place that provide environment where the individuals can follow and maintain high-quality care.

Altogether, all the processes and systems under clinical governance help in providing an umbrella of safety and quality of patient care. These systems are in place not only for the clinicians, but for every healthcare professional coming in contact with the patient. The main focus of services in the NHS has been

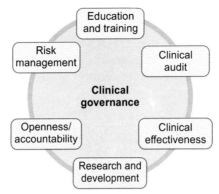

Fig. 9.1: Elements of clinical governance.[3]

shifted to patient-centred care. The various elements of clinical governance are described in Figure 9.1 and are as follows:

- Practice of evidence-based medicine and clinical effectiveness
- Research and development
- Risk management
- Clinical audit
- Education, training, and continuing professional development
- Openness or accountability
- Information management.

All these elements are based on the following principles: team work, leadership, ownership, system awareness, and communication. Of the various elements of clinical governance, the concept of risk management and clinical audit would be described in details in this chapter.

Risk Management

Over recent years, there has been a growing appreciation that a small but significant proportion of patients may experience adverse events, as a result of an error on the part of the healthcare workers, e.g. errors in the route of administration or dosage of medicines by the nurses. Sometimes, these events may prove to be serious or even life-threatening. Over the past few decades, there has been an increasing trend towards application of principles of risk management in healthcare organisations. Since small errors can result in particularly disastrous and costly adverse outcomes in both obstetrics and gynaecology, it is appropriate to review clinical risk management issues. Risk management involves the ways in which these errors can be identified, analysed, and subsequently reduced. It involves examining the various procedures, right from the beginning until their end. The various incidents and accidents are analysed to prevent their occurrence. This is based on the principle that simple system errors can result in some of the most devastating mistakes. The concept of risk management is based on the following strategies:[4]

- Identification, characterisation, and assessment of potential threats
- Assessment of the vulnerability of critical assets to specific threats
- *Determining the risk:* This involves assessment of the expected consequences of specific types of attacks on various assets
- Identifying ways for reducing those risks
- Prioritising risk reduction measures.

An educational and supportive environment, rather than a blame culture, helps in encouraging the reporting of adverse incidents. This encourages the staff to learn from the adverse outcomes. Reduction in the adverse events, which occur in healthcare institutions, helps in improving the overall quality of patient care. Within the NHS, risk is managed best within a framework, called RADICAL framework, which incorporates all elements of clinical governance. The RADICAL (Raise Awareness, Design for safety, Involvement of users, Collection and Analysis of safety data, and Learning from patient safety incidents) framework for risk management in the healthcare system is described in Flow chart 9.1.[5]

Process of Risk Management

The steps of risk management include risk identification; compilation of a risk register; risk analysis; risk treatment and risk control.

- *Risk identification:* Identification of anything which interferes with safe delivery and good-quality maternity services, requires formal processing. If something goes wrong, the clinicians can identify the risk by looking back at the series of events to identify the things that went wrong. Risks could also be identified through internal or external sources. Internal sources for identifying risk refer to risk assessment conducted in all clinical areas (wards, clinics, theatre, delivery suite, day assessment unit, etc.) as well as non-clinical areas (secretarial office, canteen, etc.). Risk assessment can also be obtained through reporting of incidents; record of complaints and claims; consultation with the staff in form of workshops, surveys, interviews and clinical audit, etc. External sources identify the risk at national level and include National Confidential Enquiries, Clinical Negligence Scheme for Trusts (CNST) standards, RCOG guidelines, NICE guidelines, protocols and visitation, National Patient Safety Agency Alerts (NPSA), postgraduate dean's specialty site visits and Care Quality Commission (CQC). Each maternity as well as gynaecology unit should have a trigger list for reporting of incidents (Tables 9.1 and 9.2). Staff must be encouraged to complete incident forms for these various triggers. To optimise the reporting of incidents, an organisation should have a culture wherein staff should be aware and motivated about reporting of adverse events. They should be aware that they would be listened to and not blamed for the adverse event. In fact, they should be provided with an accurate feedback because feedback drives motivation, which would eventually help in improvement.
- *Compilation of a risk register:* Identified risks should be entered in the risk registers, which should be preferably maintained in the clinical area of each maternity and gynaecology unit. Example of various risks, which could be

Flow chart 9.1: The RADICAL framework for the management of risk in healthcare.[5]

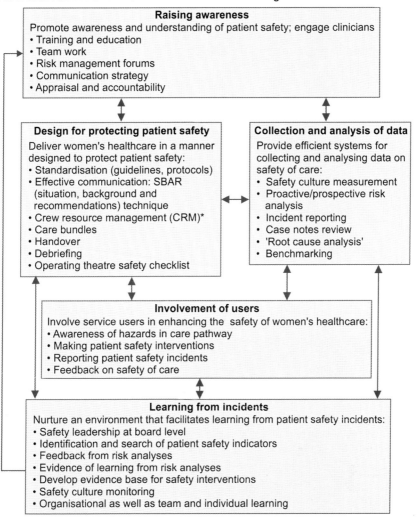

Raising awareness

Promote awareness and understanding of patient safety; engage clinicians
- Training and education
- Team work
- Risk management forums
- Communication strategy
- Appraisal and accountability

Design for protecting patient safety

Deliver women's healthcare in a manner designed to protect patient safety:
- Standardisation (guidelines, protocols)
- Effective communication: SBAR (situation, background and recommendations) technique
- Crew resource management (CRM)*
- Care bundles
- Handover
- Debriefing
- Operating theatre safety checklist

Collection and analysis of data

Provide efficient systems for collecting and analysing data on safety of care:
- Safety culture measurement
- Proactive/prospective risk analysis
- Incident reporting
- Case notes review
- 'Root cause analysis'
- Benchmarking

Involvement of users

Involve service users in enhancing the safety of women's healthcare:
- Awareness of hazards in care pathway
- Making patient safety interventions
- Reporting patient safety incidents
- Feedback on safety of care

Learning from incidents

Nurture an environment that facilitates learning from patient safety incidents:
- Safety leadership at board level
- Identification and search of patient safety indicators
- Feedback from risk analyses
- Evidence of learning from risk analyses
- Develop evidence base for safety interventions
- Safety culture monitoring
- Organisational as well as team and individual learning

*Set of training procedures for use in environments where human error can have overwhelming effects.

included in a gynaecology risk register, may include the risks identified in the care pathways for management of gynaecological emergencies, etc. However, risk registers are not merely limited to clinical issues. Non-clinical issues such as those related to breakdown of building, heating system, etc. can also be noted in the risk register. Once the risk is identified, it is graded within a standard matrix described in Table 9.3. In this matrix, the risk is scored in two ways. First one is the seriousness or consequences of risk (from being a negligible event to a catastrophic event, which can result in multiple fatalities). Various levels of severity are defined locally, with an account for the extent of harm caused to the patient and the organisation.

TABLE 9.1: Suggested trigger list for incident reporting in maternity unit.[5]

Maternal incident	Foetal/neonatal incident	Organisational incidents
• Death of the mother • Undiagnosed breech presentation • Shoulder dystocia • Blood loss >1,500 mL • Return to theatre • Eclampsia • Hysterectomy/laparotomy • Anaesthetic complications • Intensive care admission • Venous thromboembolism • Pulmonary embolism • Third-/fourth-degree perineal tears • Unsuccessful attempt at forceps or ventouse-assisted delivery • Uterine rupture • Readmission of mother	• Death of the neonate • Stillbirth >500 g • APGAR score <7 at 5 minutes • Birth trauma • Foetal laceration at the time of operative delivery • Cord pH <7.05 arterial or <7.1 venous • Neonatal seizures • Term baby admitted to neonatal unit • Undiagnosed foetal anomaly	• Unavailability of health record • Delay in responding to call for assistance • Unplanned home birth • Faulty equipment • Conflict over case management • Potential service/user complaint • Medication error • Retained swab or instrument • Hospital-acquired infection • Violation of local protocol

TABLE 9.2: Suggested trigger list for incident reporting in gynaecology unit.[5]

Clinical incident	Organisational incidents
• Damage to structures (e.g. ureter, bowel, and vessel) • Delayed or missed diagnosis (e.g. ectopic pregnancy) • Anaesthetic complications • Venous thromboembolism • Failed procedures (e.g. termination of pregnancy, sterilisation) • Unplanned intensive care admission • Omission of planned procedures (failure to insert planned intrauterine contraceptive device after a hysteroscopy) • Unexpected operative blood loss >500 mL • Moderate/severe ovarian hyperstimulation (assisted conception) • Procedure performed without consent (e.g. removal of ovaries at hysterectomy) • Unplanned return to theatre • Unplanned return to hospital within 30 days	• Delay following call for assistance • Faulty equipment • Conflict over case management • Potential service user complaint • Medication error • Retained swab or instrument • Violation of local protocol

The second score reflects the probability of the occurrence of an event (from being impossible to occur to occurring certainly). Both these scores are multiplied to reach a risk score, which helps to quantify the level of risk. Within this matrix, a risk with a score of 20 or higher is usually considered to

TABLE 9.3: Standard matrix for grading risk.

Consequences	Probability				
Severity of risk	Rare (1)	Unlikely (2)	Moderate (3)	Likely (4)	Certain (5)
Multiple fatalities (5)	5	10	15	20	25
Fatality (4)	4	8	12	16	20
Major (3)	3	6	9	12	15
Serious (2)	2	4	6	8	10
Minor (1)	1	2	3	4	5

Note: Scores obtained from the matrix can be graded as follows:
   1–3: Low risk;   4–6: Moderate risk;   8–12: High risk;   15–25: Extreme risk.

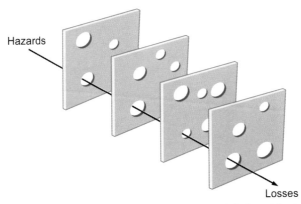

Fig. 9.2: Reason's organisational Swiss cheese model of accident causation.

represent an unacceptable risk. Residual risks exceeding a preset threshold are entered into a departmental or a directorate register. Significant risks from that register are then in turn mentioned in a hospital or trust-wide risk register. Ideally, a risk register should be in electronic format. A risk register is not a static document; it must be continually reviewed and is modified with treated or new risks. Steps must be taken for reduction of risk either by reducing the frequency of its occurrence or by reducing its severity.

- *Risk analysis*: Once the risks have been identified, they are noted in the risk register, following which they are assigned a risk score as previously described (Table 9.3). This helps in identifying those risks, which require detailed investigation and immediate action for correction. The incident must be investigated using the Reason's organisational 'Swiss cheese' model of accident causation (Fig. 9.2). This model illustrates that there are many layers of defence between hazards to accidents. Alignment of flaws in each of the layers allows the accident to occur. This model has been adopted by the NPSA and used as the 'fishbone tool' for root cause analysis. Fishbone diagrams (Fig. 9.3) are often used by the NPSA for identifying the contributory factors.[6]

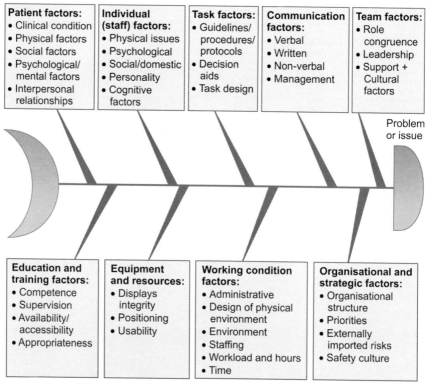

Fig. 9.3: Fishbone diagram for root cause analysis.

It helps to categorise the potential sources of defects or the root causes. Various components of a fishbone are as follows:
- *Head of the fish*: Effect or the outcome
- *Horizontal branches*: Causes (various causes can be divided into non-service processes such as methods, materials, people, equipment, technique, environment, and service processes such as policy, procedures, plan, and people)
- Sub-branches: Reasons.
- *Risk treatment*: This is a process involving selection and implementation of measures for modifying the risk. Various methods for risk treatment include elimination, substitution, reduction, and acceptance. Selection of an appropriate method depends on factors such as risk rating and resource implications. Based on this, an action plan is devised and approval is taken from the management regarding this plan. An important factor to be kept in mind is that even after the implementation of this action plan, some residual risk may remain. This residual risk must always be documented and reviewed.
- *Risk control*: Following the appropriate analysis of risk and risk treatment, measures must be put in place for controlling the risk. Selection of the appropriate treatment plan is dependent on the risk rating. Lessons learned from the identification and treatment of risk should be shared with the

healthcare professionals in other parts of the hospital or trust through several routes such as multidisciplinary team meetings, ward meetings, safety alerts, newsletters, and intranet and educational meetings. Both the NPSA and the RCOG have communication channels which can be used for this purpose.

Clinical Audit

Definition

The NICE has defined clinical audit as '*a quality improvement process that seeks to improve patient care and outcomes through systematic review of care against explicit criteria and the implementation of change. Aspects of the structure, processes, and outcomes of care are selected and systematically evaluated against explicit criteria. Where indicated, changes are implemented at an individual, team, or service level and further monitoring is used to confirm improvement in healthcare delivery.*[7] Audit is the process of quality improvement of the healthcare services, thereby improving the overall quality of life. It aims at improving the patient care and outcome by assessing, evaluating, and improving the care of the patients.[8] This is achieved through the systematic review of care against set criteria. Based on the findings of the review, the changes are identified and implemented. Where indicated, the identified changes are implemented and monitored at different levels to confirm if these changes result in an improvement towards the delivery of healthcare services. An audit, therefore, helps in highlighting those areas where improvement is required in healthcare delivery. This eventually helps in safeguarding high quality of clinical care for patients. Difference between audit and research has been described in Table 9.4.[9]

TABLE 9.4: Difference between audit and research.

Characteristic	Research	Audit
Definition	• It is theory-driven, and discovers and defines the right thing to do to help improve knowledge	• It is practice-based and determines whether the right thing is being done in order to improve healthcare services
Aims	• Aims for generalisation of the findings • Aims to find out the best practice	• It is never possible to generalise the findings because each report deals with an individual situation • Aims to find how close is current practice to best practice?
Special feature	• It is a one-off project where each project stands alone	• It is an ongoing process and involves a cyclical series of reviews
Methodology	• Collection of complex and unique data by specific researchers • May involve an experimental treatment or placebo	• Collection of routine data carried out by members of the multidisciplinary team • Never involves an experimental treatment or placebo

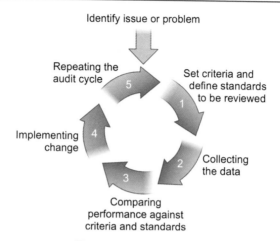

Fig. 9.4: The audit cycle.

Steps of Audit Cycle

A typical audit cycle is described in Figure 9.4 and comprises the following steps:[9]

1. *Initial needs assessment*: The audit cycle comprises an initial needs assessment where the requirements of the department or section or individual are determined and the actual audit itself is determined.
2. *Identification of standards*: It is essential to identify the standards, once the topic for audit has been decided, against which the audit will be compared. For this, the criteria for the current best practice need to be determined. These can be national standards or clinical guidelines determined by the national bodies or comparisons can even be made within the department. Common standards include: NICE guidance, Royal College Guidance, guidelines by the national service frameworks, local policies, etc.
3. *Data collection and analysis*: Once the standards have been set, data, which is to be collected, needs to be identified. The methodology for data collection as well as who is going to collect the data is decided, following which the data collection is undertaken. The sample size and prospective or retrospective collection of data needs to be decided.

   The collected data is then analysed wherein the actual performance within the department is compared with the set standard. In case the results show that the set standards are not being followed, the possible reasons behind this discrepancy are explored.
4. *Comparing current practice with the standard and presenting recommendations*: The data collected represents actual performance within the department. This is then compared with the set standard. Assessment of how well the standards are met is carried out. The results are then presented to the relevant multidisciplinary teams within the organisation. In case the standards are not met, the reasons behind this are identified. From this analysis, recommendations for further improvements or implementation

of changes are made. Finally, an action plan is developed, agreed and implemented in order to bring actual practice closer to the standard.

5. *Re-audit*: Subsequently after the intervention has been implemented, new data is collected to determine the impact. This data is again compared with the standard to establish if there was an improvement in practice. Finally, to assess how effectively these recommendations have been implemented, a re-audit is suggested in the future.

OSCE STATION 1: DESIGNING A PROTOCOL FOR THE IDENTIFICATION AND MANAGEMENT OF FOETAL GROWTH RESTRICTION IN YOUR ANTENATAL CARE WARD AND DEMONSTRATING THE SUCCESS OF YOUR PROTOCOL

Candidate's Instructions

Foetal growth restriction or FGR, remains an important cause of foetal and neonatal morbidity and mortality in the UK. You have been requested to produce a protocol for properly managing this condition in your unit and to demonstrate the success of your protocol. The task is for 12 minutes (inclusive of 2 minutes of reading time). You have 10 minutes to tell the examiner about the protocol. You shall be awarded marks for the following tasks:

Candidate's tasks:

- Producing a protocol for properly managing FGR in your unit to reduce the associated morbidity and mortality
- Demonstrating the success of your protocol.

These tasks cover the domains as discussed next.

Core Clinical Skills Domains

Core clinical skills domains tested:

- Patient safety
- Communication with patients
- Information gathering
- Application of knowledge.

Module Tested

The modules tested in this station are Module 1 or 'Teaching' and Module 5 or 'Maternal Medicine'.

EXAMINER'S INSTRUCTIONS AND STRUCTURED MARK SHEET

The examiner will mark the candidate on the basis of various tasks, which are allotted to the candidate. Out of a total score of 20, the examiner can award a maximum of 20 marks, which are distributed between various candidate tasks as shown next. Each candidate task must be globally scored by the examiner.

The process of designing a protocol involves the following steps described next.

Identification of the Standards

The standards, which would be used as the benchmark for comparison, need to be determined. The standards can be determined through MedLine® search/literature review from the following sources:
- National Institute for Health and Care Excellence guidelines
- Royal College of Obstetricians and Gynaecologists guidelines
- Cochrane reviews
- Meta-analyses
- Randomised controlled trials
- Other types of studies
- Data to be collected from other units
- Textbooks
- Opinions of respected colleagues.

When undertaking this search, the candidate needs to focus on the relevant aspects of the protocol. For example, in this case, the candidate's search would focus on the known causes of FGR and the populations at risk, the incidence, diagnosis, and management (monitoring, mode of delivery, and timing of delivery). Candidates should be aware about the limitations of the various types of evidence.

Marking Scheme

0	1	2	3	4
Fail	Borderline		Pass	

Data Collection: Designing a Pro forma to Collect Information

- The pro forma must be designed so that it can identify the at-risk groups. Once the candidate has defined the standards, he/she needs to design a pro forma containing the following information:

Definition of FGR

Birth weight is lower than the 10th percentile of the average for the particular gestational age.

Defining the High-risk Groups

- The high risk groups for the development of intrauterine growth restriction (IUGR) are described in Table 9.5.
- Need to decide the sample size
- Need to decide the type of audit—prospective or retrospective. Candidate must be familiar with the advantages and disadvantages of each type.
- If required, candidate must consult the audit unit to help him to design the pro forma and also to help calculate the power for the audit. This helps in confirming that the outcome measures are statistically acceptable.

TABLE 9.5: Risk factors for the development of IUGR.

Maternal factors	Foetal factors	Placental factors
• Constitutionally small mothers • Maternal undernutrition • Tobacco smoking, excessive alcohol intake, drug abuse during pregnancy, etc. • Chronic placental insufficiency due to pre-eclampsia, chronic hypertension, renal disease, connective tissue disorders, gestational diabetes, etc. • Maternal consumption of drugs including hydantoin, coumarin, etc. • Maternal hypoxia (pulmonary diseases, cyanotic congenital heart disease, etc.) • Endocrine disorders (e.g. diabetic nephropathy, hyperthyroidism, and Addison's disease)	• Multiple pregnancy • Congenital malformations (congenital heart disease, renal agenesis, etc.) • Chromosomal abnormalities (trisomy 21, 13, 18, 16, etc.) • Intrauterine foetal infections (rubella, CMV, herpes, toxoplasmosis, tuberculosis, syphilis, etc.)	*Uteroplacental insufficiency*: • Unexplained • Essential hypertension • Pre-eclampsia • Chronic renal disease • Elevated maternal AFP *Fetoplacental insufficiency*: • Single umbilical artery • Velamentous insertion of cord • Placental haemangioma *Abnormal placentation*: • Abruptio placentae • Placenta praevia • Placenta accreta *Placental abnormalities*: • Placental thrombosis • Placental infection • Chorioamnionitis, placental cysts, etc.

(IUGR: intrauterine growth restriction; AFP: alpha-fetoprotein; CMV: cytomegalovirus)

Causes of FGR

- Low maternal weight gain during pregnancy
- Extremes of maternal body mass index (BMI <20 kg/m² or BMI >25 kg/m²)
- Cigarette smoking
- Alcohol or drug abuse
- Genetic factors
- Short maternal stature
- Primiparity
- Maternal age more than equal to 35 years, with a further increase in those greater than 40 years old
- African American or Indian/Asian ethnicity
- Social deprivation
- A short (<6 months) or long (>60 months) inter-pregnancy interval
- Heavy vaginal bleeding in the first trimester
- Foetal factors: Infections, chromosomal abnormalities, etc.
- Placental insufficiency: Pre-eclampsia.

Diagnosis of FGR

- *Ultrasound biometry*: Head circumference/abdominal circumference (HC/AC) ratio or femur length/abdominal circumference (FL/AC) ratio, and ultrasound estimated foetal weight.

- *Invasive tests*: Foetal karyotyping, screening for congenital infections.
- *Biophysical tests*: Nonstress test, biophysical profile, amniotic fluid volume, ultrasound Doppler flow velocimetry [umbilical artery S/D (systolic/diastolic) ratio, resistance index, pulsatility index; middle cerebral artery studies; venous Doppler reversal of blood flow in inferior vena cava, ductus venosus, and umbilical vein at the end of diastole], foetal cardiotocography, etc.

Management of FGR

- Identification and treatment of the underlying cause
- Rest in left lateral position
- Daily foetal movement count
- Prescription of low-dose aspirin
- Foetal surveillance during the antenatal period
- Deciding the time for delivery by weighing the risk of foetal demise due to delayed intervention against the risk of long-term disabilities resulting from preterm delivery due to early intervention.[10]
- The two main parameters for deciding the optimal time of delivery include results on various foetal surveillance techniques and gestational age.[11]

Marking Scheme

0	1	2	3	4
Fail	Borderline		Pass	

Analysis of the Data and Presentation to the Stakeholders

- Once the data has been collected, it needs to be analysed and presented to all stakeholders.
- Representatives from various stakeholders, which need to be involved, include the following:
  - General practitioner (GP)
  - Nurses, those belonging to ward/theatre, radiology/ultrasound unit
  - Midwives
  - Consultant obstetricians.

Marking Scheme

0	1	2	3	4
Fail	Borderline		Pass	

Discussion and Implementation of Recommendations

- Recommendations must be discussed, agreed upon, and implemented.
- If the outcome measures are statistically significant, the method needs to be implemented in clinical practice.

Dissemination of Protocol and its Implementation

- The protocol must be circulated amongst various stakeholders for comments.
- The comments must be collated and the protocol modified as appropriate
- Date of implementation needs to be decided upon and the protocol needs to be implemented with the support of clinical director on the predesigned date.
- The protocol must be communicated to all users including GPs, healthcare professionals in A&E (accident & emergency) unit, the labour unit, obstetric unit, and the ultrasound unit. It must also be made available in all units and GP surgeries.

Marking Scheme

0	1	2	3	4
Fail	Borderline		Pass	

Re-audit: Demonstration of Success of Protocol

- Following a well-defined time frame, a re-audit needs to be conducted
- After a defined period of implementation (determined by the number of cases required for an effective audit), the following outcome measures need to be evaluated:
  - Diagnosis of cases of IUGR
  - Management: Timing of delivery and the mode of delivery
  - Missed cases of IUGR babies
  - Delivered cases of IUGR babies
  - Intrauterine growth restriction babies requiring admission to the neonatal intensive care unit (NICU)
  - Intrauterine growth restriction babies suffering from both short-term and long-term disability
  - Mortality.
- Dissemination of the audit outcomes to members of the unit and discussion of recommendations.

Marking Scheme

0	1	2	3	4
Fail	Borderline		Pass	

Total score: /20

DISCUSSION

Issues

In such kind of stations, it is important for the candidate to read the task carefully and realise that there are two parts to the question: drawing up a clinical protocol and conducting an audit. All ST5 level trainees are expected to be familiar with conducting a clinical audit as well as drawing up of protocols, which are important components of clinical governance.

In this station, when drawing up a protocol for the identification and management of cases of FGR, the candidate's search must focus on the known causes of FGR and the populations at risk, the incidence of FGR, and its diagnosis and management (monitoring and timing of delivery). Based on this information, the candidate should be able to draw up a pro forma for identification of at-risk groups, methods for diagnosing the cases of FGR when it develops, monitoring the foetuses, and deciding the time and mode of delivery.

Once the pro forma has been designed, it must be disseminated amongst various stake holders. Following the discussion between various stakeholders, the recommendations must be reached which must be then implemented in the various units. To be able to analyse if a particular protocol is demonstrating a benefit to the unit, the data related to outcome needs to be analysed. The candidates should be aware of the following situations: ensuring that everyone in the unit buys into the recommendations; convincing the consultants in case they refuse to accept the recommendations; methods for disseminating the results of the audit to the various stakeholders; and implementing the protocol without marginalising colleagues.

Pitfalls

Going straight to the audit part and failing to address the protocol is likely to result in failure. The candidate must carefully read the question to understand what they are really required to do.

Variations

Designing a protocol for audit could be related to any of the condition which is not been properly managed in the department. However, the process of designing a protocol and conducting an audit more or less remains the same. Audit may also be required for issues holding high priority for one's department/trust or hospital, e.g. areas with a high volume of work load or those having a high rate of complications.

OSCE STATION 2: SETTING UP A RISK MANAGEMENT TEAM IN YOUR UNIT FOR IDENTIFICATION OF MISSED CASES OF ECTOPIC PREGNANCY

Candidate's Instructions

The clinical lead in your obstetric unit has noted an increase in the number of cases of ectopic pregnancy, which are wrongly managed. You are the ST5 posted in this unit and have been asked to assist in setting up a risk management team in your unit for the identification of cases of ectopic pregnancy where the diagnosis was either missed or delayed. This is a structured viva for 12 minutes (inclusive of 2 minutes of reading time). You have 10 minutes to answer the examiner's questions. You shall be awarded marks for the following tasks:

Candidate's tasks:

- What is a risk management team?
- What is the risk management team composed of?
- Describe the procedure of risk management in this case
- What are the responsibilities of the risk management team.

These tasks cover the domains as discussed next.

Core Clinical Skills Domains

Core clinical skills domains tested:

- Patient safety
- Information gathering
- Application of knowledge.

Module Tested

The modules tested in this station are Module 1 or 'Teaching' and Module 12 or 'Early Pregnancy Care.'

EXAMINER'S INSTRUCTIONS AND STRUCTURED MARK SHEET

The examiner will mark the candidate on the basis of various tasks, which are allotted to the candidate. Out of a total score of 20, the examiner can award a maximum of 20 marks, which are distributed between various candidate tasks as shown next. Each candidate task must be globally scored by the examiner.

Definition of a Risk Management Team

- Risk management is increasingly being recognised as an important component of clinical governance.
- Risk management is more so important in the light of the rising cost of litigation in obstetrics and gynaecology, with the specialty comprising nearly 60% of the NHS litigation bill.
- The Clinical Negligence Scheme for Trusts requires all units to have risk management teams.
- Once the team has been established, this information must be disseminated to the unit through meetings and other kinds of forum.
- Members of risk management teams must be seen to work in collaboration with all aspects of the services provided within the team.

Marking Scheme

0	1	2	3	4	5
Fail	Borderline		Pass		

Composition of the Risk Management Team

- Within each unit, there should be a risk manager working within the risk management team with the aim of minimising risk.
- Membership of the risk management team must reflect the multidisciplinary nature of patient care within the unit and must work in collaboration with all aspects of the services provided within the team.
- The team must include a midwife or nurse, obstetricians (trainees and consultants), and an anaesthetist.
- The members of the team should have an interest in risk management. They must preferably be educated regarding the importance of risk management as a means of improving healthcare services.

Marking Scheme

0	1	2	3	4
Fail	Borderline		Pass	

Process of Risk Management

- *Risk identification*: This involves looking back to identify what went wrong? Risk is identified through internal and external sources. Internal sources in this case would include wards, clinics, delivery suites, and ultrasound units. Risks are obtained through reporting of incidents, and record of complaints and claims. Issues, which the risk management team is required to explore further, need to be identified. The risks and previous complaints identified through the above-mentioned methods must have been entered into a risk register from where they can be collated and reviewed.
  - Why were the cases of ectopic pregnancy missed?
  - Were ultrasound facilities not available?
  - Were ultrasound technicians not available?
  - Was there lack of expertise in diagnosing the cases of ectopic pregnancy?
- Staff is encouraged to complete incident forms for various triggers.
- *Compilation of a risk register*: Incident forms related to mismanagement of cases of ectopic pregnancy, which had been compiled in a risk register, need to be reviewed.
- *Risk analysis*: Once the risk is identified, it is graded with a standard matrix, following which they are assigned a risk score. This helps in the identification of risks or incidents, which require an in-depth investigation or an immediate action for correction.
- *Risk treatment*: An action plan is devised. This is a process involving selection and implementation of measures for modifying the risk factors which led to the misdiagnosis of the cases of ectopic pregnancy. Root cause analysis is carried out using a fishbone model.
- *Risk control*: Measures must be put in place for controlling these risks. The results must also be shared with the other healthcare professionals through multidisciplinary meetings, ward meetings, newsletters, educational meetings, etc.

Marking Scheme

0	1	2	3	4	5	6
Fail		Borderline		Pass		

Responsibilities of the Team

- The responsibilities of the team must be clearly defined.
- The team should aim at identifying the risk management issues within the unit.
- Guidelines must be set regarding the management of various issues and minimising the risk management issues within the unit.
- The risk management team performs the following roles:
  - Ensuring that complaints are dealt with rapidly and early
  - Identification of the potential problems at an early stage
  - Dealing with the identified problems at an early stage
  - Educating the members of staff in those areas where weaknesses are identified in their practices.
- Setting up a register for reporting different incidents so that various risk-management issues could be identified.
- Setting up a process set in place to deal with any deficiencies in the unit.
- Clearly defining the role of the risk management team within the unit.
- Setting up the channels of two-way communication between the team, members of staff, and management.
- Making efforts to ensure that the staff in the unit does not perceive the team as a fault-finding and blame-placing team. Rather this team must be perceived as one whose role is constructive, aiming for a risk-free service within the unit.

Marking Scheme

0	1	2	3	4	5
Fail		Borderline		Pass	

Total score: /20

DISCUSSION

Issues

As a ST5 trainee, the candidate is expected to demonstrate a working knowledge regarding the principles of risk management. Risk management comprises of three main areas: identification, analysis, and treatment and control. The candidates mainly need to ask themselves three kinds of questions:
- What went wrong?
- How did it go wrong?
- What can be done to stop it from going wrong again?

Defined problems/errors must prompt a clinical incident report in the NHS. Various clinical incidence reports are collated into a database so that they can be analysed. The analysis helps in the identification of trends, which has resulted in errors. These could be the problems associated with the clinical system or the problems associated with the individuals and these need to be addressed. Blame should not be allocated to an individual or a system. Serious incidents or trends need to be analysed in details. This helps in producing a series of recommendations for future so that the problems can be identified and tackled.

Pitfalls

The process of risk management is different from that of an audit. Talking about the steps of audit on such kind of stations can be considered as a potential mistake.

Variations

Different risk management tasks could be related to various triggers in both obstetrics and gynaecology units as described in Tables 9.1 and 9.2, respectively.

OSCE STATION 3: CONSTRUCTING AN AUDIT TO REDUCE THE MORBIDITY AND MORTALITY RELATED TO ECTOPIC PREGNANCY

Candidate's Instructions

A copy of an algorithm that is used in the early pregnancy assessment unit is supplied. This protocol was instituted in order to reduce the mortality and morbidity associated with the cases of ectopic pregnancy.

You are required to design an audit to determine how well the protocol is being followed in the EPU to reduce the rate of mortality and morbidity related to ectopic pregnancy.

The task is for 12 minutes (inclusive of 2 minutes of reading time). You have 10 minutes to answer the examiner's questions. You shall be awarded marks for the following tasks:

Candidate's tasks:

- Discuss with the examiner how you would design an audit to ascertain how well this protocol is being adhered to.
- Discuss the factors you would take into consideration while designing the audit.
- What steps you would take if the audit revealed that overall compliance was poor?

These tasks cover the domains as discussed next.

Core Clinical Skills Domains

Core clinical skills domains tested:

- Patient safety
- Application of knowledge.

Module Tested

The modules tested in this station are Module 1 or 'Teaching' and Module 12 or 'Early Pregnancy Care'.

EXAMINER'S INSTRUCTIONS AND STRUCTURED MARK SHEET

The examiner will mark the candidate on the basis of various tasks which are allotted to the candidate. Out of a total score of 20, the examiner can award a maximum of 20 marks, which are distributed between various candidate tasks as shown next. Each candidate task must be globally scored by the examiner. The candidate is not being asked to comment on or criticise the protocol as such. Candidates need to cover the following areas of discussion and can be encouraged using specific questions to answer in the correct direction if they do not mention them spontaneously:

- Designing an audit to address the question
- Discussing the factors they would take into consideration
- Discussing how you would use the results.

Designing the Audit

Identification of Standards

- Determining the best practice using evidence-based medicine (RCOG/national guidelines) for the management of cases of ectopic pregnancy
- Consumer interaction or expectations
- Previous audit findings
- Encouraging all stakeholders to make comments
- Defining the standards for the audit as follows:
    - Definition of extrauterine pregnancies
    - Prevalence of ectopic pregnancies
    - Causes of ectopic pregnancy
    - Diagnosis of ectopic pregnancy
    - Management of ectopic pregnancies.
- Defining the high-risk group as follows:
    - Previous history of infection (pelvic inflammatory disease or sexually transmitted disease) with *Chlamydia trachomatis* or *Neisseria gonorrhoea.*
    - Previous history of salpingitis or tuberculosis
    - Previous history of ectopic pregnancies
    - Promiscuous behaviour or having multiple sexual partners
    - Using intrauterine contraceptive device
    - Previous history of tubal surgery (including tubal reconstructive surgery, tubectomy, etc.)
    - Previous history of treatment for infertility
    - History of endometriosis and pelvic scar tissue (pelvic adhesions).

Marking Scheme

0	1	2	3	4	5
Fail		Borderline		Pass	

Data Collection (Designing a Pro forma to Collect Information) and Data Analysis

- Determining the sample size
- Establishing a data sheet or pro forma to identify patients' course of illness
- The course of illness would be based on the clinical presentation, diagnosis, and management plans.
- Defining the outcome criteria
- Identifying missing data and eliminating bias
- Identifying key failures in following the algorithm
- Deciding whether the audit would be prospective or retrospective and the inherent problems associated with both types.

Use of Audit Results to Reframe Recommendations

- The following outcome measures need to be analysed:
  - Diagnosis
  - Treatment—tubal conservation and non-tubal removal
  - Missed cases of ectopic pregnancy
  - Number of cases of ruptured ectopics
  - Cases of ectopic pregnancy requiring blood transfusion.
- Admission into hospital and mortality rate also needs to be analysed
- Audit outcomes to be disseminated to the members of the unit followed by the discussion of recommendations
- Implementation of changes identified
- Completing the audit cycle by conducting a re-audit
- Deciding the time for repeating the audit.

Marking Scheme

0	1	2	3	4	5
Fail		Borderline		Pass	

Factors to be taken into Consideration while Designing the Audit

Clinical Presentation

This would include the following:
- History—pain, irregular vaginal bleeding, and vaginal discharge
- Amenorrhoea
- Shoulder-tip pain
- Features of anaemia
- Tenderness (abdomen and cervical, especially excitation tenderness)
- Adnexal mass; fullness in the pouch of Douglas.

Investigations

- Urinary pregnancy test
- Beta-human chorionic gonadotropin (β-hCG) levels
- Full blood count
- Group and save/cross-match
- Serial measurements of β-hCG
- Ultrasound—transvaginal or abdominal.

Treatment

- Expectant management
- Surgery
- Laparotomy or laparoscopy
- Salpingectomy, salpingotomy, milking out the tubal contents
- Medical management, e.g. methotrexate (intramuscular)
- Follow-up after conservative (tube-preserving) management.

Marking Scheme

0	1	2	3	4	5
Fail		Borderline		Pass	

Steps to be taken if Audit Results Reveal Poor Compliance

- Feedback of the results after analysis must be provided back to the staff.
- May require speaking to the GPs or holding meetings with the various stakeholders.
- Consider any necessary organisational changes, which need to be implemented for improving or allowing compliance.
- New changes should be implemented in such a way that the concerned issued are handled strongly, without putting a blame on the individuals involved.
- Need to decide the method for achieving consistent implementation after involving the stakeholders.

Marking Scheme

0	1	2	3	4	5
Fail		Borderline		Pass	

Total score: /20

DISCUSSION

Issues

This station is designed to test the candidate's understanding of audit. The algorithm or protocol is relatively immaterial in this case. It is not the protocol that is being criticised but the adherence to the protocol that is being tested. The examiner will expect the candidate to go through the steps of an audit cycle.

If the examiner has to prompt the candidate then the marking will be reflected accordingly.

Pitfalls

The major pitfall is lack of understanding in the audit process and spending time in criticising the protocol. All UK trainees are expected to undertake some form of audit during their postings and this is the place to learn how to do it. The candidates must be aware about the audit pro forma or data sheets that need to be produced. They also need to be aware regarding whether the audit should be done on the basis of sample size or a specified time frame. The candidates must also be aware about the two types of audit: retrospective and the prospective, and the advantages and disadvantages which are associated with both. This usually depends upon the frequency of the condition under consideration. For early pregnancy problems, it may be useful to conduct an audit based on the sample size. On the other hand, in case of an audit of a procedure (e.g. water births, breech vaginal delivery, foetal scalp blood sampling, etc.) it may be useful to conduct an audit using a fixed time frame. Most audits should be done prospectively because there is a risk of losing cases with a retrospective audit. This may eventually alter the ultimate outcome.

Variations

It is important for the candidates to be familiar with the steps of audit. For this it may be useful for them if they have undertaken an audit previously within their own organisation. They must be aware about the following steps to be adhered while conducting an audit: deciding the audit title based on the scope and objectives of the condition under consideration; reviewing the current practice; deciding the preferred best practice; designing the audit methodology or pro forma (audit tool); method for collection and analysis of data; and formulation of recommendations and implementation of an action plan. The final step, which involves closing the audit loop, includes re-audit. All the previously mentioned steps are repeated again in order to close the loop. After some time has passed for the intervention to take effect, new data is collected to determine the impact produced by implementation of the changes. This is then again compared with the set standard to establish if this has resulted in an improvement in practice.

Each of the above-described steps of audit can serve as an individual station and candidates can encounter any of these during the examination. Thus they need to be familiar with all the steps of an audit cycle.

OSCE STATION 4: CLINICAL GOVERNANCE (HYPOXIC ISCHAEMIC ENCEPHALOPATHY IN A BABY)

The case of Mrs Susan Adams is to be discussed at the monthly Governance Meeting. Mrs Adams is a 28-year-old woman, delivered by the midwife. The baby who was born sustained an hypoxic ischaemic encephalopathy (HIE) after a difficult vaginal delivery, where the midwife particularly faced difficulty during delivery of shoulders. You are the ST5 registrar posted in this ward and you have been asked to organise a feedback session on management of shoulder dystocia. This will involve all grades of doctors in the obstetrics department as well as the theatre and the healthcare staff belonging to related departments (paediatrics and anaesthesia).

Candidate's Instructions

You are about to explain to the Clinical Lead for Governance how you plan to approach the session. The Clinical Lead has been asked not to interrupt you over the allocated time. You have to refer to the index case so as to cover the basic principles of management related to shoulder dystocia. The task is for 12 minutes (inclusive of 2 minutes of reading time). You have 10 minutes to discuss the situation with the examiner. This task is a structured discussion assessing the candidate's ability for carrying out the following tasks:

Candidate's tasks:

- How do you plan to approach the session?
- Highlight how problems occur and how to avoid them
- Refer to the index case
- What recommendations would you make on reviewing this case?

Case Study

This was Mrs Adam's first pregnancy and it was a planned one. She had been diagnosed as a case of gestational diabetes during this pregnancy. Her booking BMI was 32 kg/m^2 and her fasting blood glucose levels were raised. She has been receiving insulin throughout her antenatal period in view of her raised blood sugar values. A glucose tolerance test during the last antenatal visit was found to be within the normal limits.

   She did not appear to have any antenatal problems apart from an episode of reduced foetal movements at 33 weeks, which had resolved spontaneously. She was seen regularly alternating the visits between the midwife and the hospital antenatal clinic throughout the pregnancy. All her observations were normal. In view of her gestational diabetes, a growth scan was arranged at 34 weeks' gestation, which showed a normally grown foetus, with a cephalic presentation. She presented to the antenatal clinic at term with regular uterine contractions at 7:00 pm. The vaginal examination during this visit revealed a partially effaced cervix which was 7–8 cm dilated.

   A cardiotocograph was undertaken and this was normal. Consequently, she was transferred to the labour ward. One hour later, at 8:30 pm, she became fully dilated and fully effaced and was having good uterine contractions. By 9:00 pm, she was bearing down. Soon the baby's head was delivered. The midwife who was attending the patient was still undergoing training. The senior midwife was busy attending another patient and was taking a breech vaginal delivery. However, the midwife with Mrs Adams was unable to deliver the baby's body completely. The baby appeared to be stuck at the shoulder.

The midwife panicked and struggled for nearly 10 minutes before calling the ST5 on duty in the labour ward. On arriving, the ST5 summoned anaesthetist, paediatrician, and labour ward coordinator. The baby was delivered at 10:30 pm with an APGAR score of 4 and weight of 4.8 kg. Resuscitation was attempted by the paediatric team, and the baby was admitted in the NICU after the consultant paediatrician had discussed the situation with the parents. The diagnosis of HIE due to chronic hypoxia was made.

On reflection, it appears that the situation was not handled efficiently by the midwife. Also, more importance was given to the maternal gestational diabetes and less on the probable macrosomia in the baby which possibly led to shoulder dystocia, resulting in the delay in the baby's delivery. The risk of acidosis or HIE is very low when the head to body delivery interval is less than 5 minutes.[12] The respective risk increases as the head to body delivery interval increases.

The following props have been provided to the candidate: dummy pelvis and doll.

The candidate's tasks cover the domains as discussed next.

Core Clinical Skills Domains

Core clinical skills domains tested:
- Patient safety
- Communication with colleagues
- Application of knowledge.

Module Tested

The modules tested in this station are Module 1 or 'Teaching' and Module 7 or 'Management of Delivery'.

EXAMINER'S INSTRUCTIONS AND STRUCTURED MARK SHEET

The examiner will mark the candidate on the basis of various tasks, which are allotted to the candidate. Out of a total score of 20, the examiner can award a maximum of 20 marks, which are distributed between various candidate tasks as shown next. Each candidate task must be globally scored by the examiner. As part of the action plan, the candidate (as an ST5) has been asked to organise a feedback session on the management of shoulder dystocia. This will involve all grades of doctors in the department as well as the midwives and labour coordinators. Your task is to explain the background to the session and the possible complications of diabetic pregnancies, with special emphasis on shoulder dystocia. In particular, you need to highlight how shoulder dystocia can arise and how can you manage this complication.

Approaching the Session

- The candidate demonstrates that he/she has reviewed the case in details and recognises the need to involve all the midwives, theatre staff, anaesthetists, and paediatricians as well as junior doctors and consultants.

- The candidate shows understanding regarding the requirement to tackle difficult issues with the help of colleagues and that they are capable of working under pressure.
- The competent candidate should be able to cooperatively communicate with the governance lead clarifying the probable cause of the injury.
- This task focuses on the candidate's capability of formulating a strategy to deliver a teaching session, which would also help in evaluating the candidate's teaching skills.
- The competent candidate will begin with the purpose of the session and its importance.
- The candidate must demonstrate clear understanding of the cause for the session in terms of avoidable damage to the baby due to shoulder dystocia. Candidate should explain that this situation should not have occurred and is most likely linked to the delay involved in the delivery of baby's shoulders.
- Before conducting the tutorial, the candidate needs to adopt a structured and comprehensive approach to the task and must identify the following details:
  - Understanding of the aims and objectives of the tutorial
  - The knowledge level of the attendees
  - Creating an outline plan for this task, including who would form the audience, the place where the training should take place, and a suitable time to ensure good attendance.
- The candidate needs to ensure that the teaching standard is appropriate for all levels of staff and all professional groups and must demonstrate a detailed understanding of the topic they are teaching.
- They need to cover the basic principles related to shoulder dystocia.
- They must identify the various risk factors related to shoulder dystocia.
- They should adopt a logical and organised approach while demonstrating various manoeuvres for the management of shoulder dystocia using the provided tutorial props (dummy pelvis and doll).

Marking Scheme

0	1	2	3	4	5	6
Fail		Borderline		Pass		

Highlighting the Occurrence of Problems and Method of Avoiding

- This task also evaluates the candidate's comprehension regarding investigation of a critical incident and their capability for forming an action plan following a root cause analysis of the event.
- A root cause analysis helps in identifying whether there is a problem with one individual who may require training or support with a particular aspect of their clinical skills, or there is a systematic problem associated with the processes relating to management of cases of shoulder dystocia (e.g. sufficient infrastructure is not in place).

- The root cause analysis will also help in identifying the likely problems related to the system and the processes. For example, in this case inadequate training of the trainee midwives and the nursing staff may be responsible for the adverse event.
- The candidate needs to understand that the aim of this session is not to assign blame on a single individual, rather to inspire learning from adverse events.
- A root cause analysis may help in recognising that there is a risk that many members of the multidisciplinary team may not have sufficient understanding regarding the detailed issues related to the management of shoulder dystocia. Hence, all healthcare personnel must be involved in this training session.
- Main factors which may have affected the patient outcome in this case include the following:
  - Patient's high BMI complicated the application of manoeuvres by the trainee midwife.
  - Concerns were more around the mother (e.g. monitoring the blood glucose levels) rather than the foetus (failure to anticipate the difficult delivery of a macrosomic baby).
  - Shoulder dystocia is an emergency situation that is usually covered in the 'drills and skills' tutorials. This tutorial had probably not been attended by the trainee midwife.
  - Failure to realise that the woman had several predisposing factors for shoulder dystocia including gestational diabetes mellitus, raised BMI of mother, and large baby.
  - Proper monitoring of head to body delivery interval was not done. The candidate needs to emphasise that it is important that someone keeps watch on the time and shouts out after each 30 seconds so that the people involved are well aware of the time that has passed. The urgency for the delivery of the baby's body is related to the fact that the cord pH drops at the rate of 0.04/min.
- The candidate needs to highlight the fact that the management of shoulder dystocia needs to be preferably done within 5 minutes of the delivery of the foetal head in order to prevent irreversible foetal injury.[12]
- The candidate needs to explain the mnemonic, HELPERR to be used while managing the cases of shoulder dystocia (Table 9.6).[13]

Marking Scheme

0	1	2	3	4	5	6
Fail		Borderline		Pass		

Referring to the Index Case

- The candidate's tasks make it very clear to the candidate that they are required to refer to the index case who has several predisposing factors for shoulders dystocia including gestational diabetes mellitus, raised maternal

TABLE 9.6: Mnemonic HELPERR for describing initial management in the cases of shoulder dystocia.

H	Call for help (anaesthetist, paediatrician, and labour ward coordinator)
E	Evaluate for episiotomy (if she has not had an episiotomy, it may be worth performing one)
L	Legs [the McRoberts manoeuvre (Figs. 9.5A and B): patient's legs are hyperflexed at the hips and flexed at the knee]
P	Suprapubic pressure (continuous or intermittent suprapubic external pressure behind the anterior shoulder, Fig. 9.6)
E	*Enter the pelvis manoeuvres (internal rotation):* • Rubin II manoeuvre (approach anterior foetal shoulder from its posterior aspect in order to adduct the shoulder, i.e. reduce the biacromial diameters and rotate to the oblique, Fig. 9.7) • Wood's screw manoeuvre: Approaching the posterior foetal shoulder from its anterior aspect and gently rotating towards the symphysis (Fig. 9.8) • Reverse Wood's screw manoeuvre: Approaching the posterior shoulder from its posterior aspect and attempt to dislodge in the opposite direction (Fig. 9.9)
R	Remove the posterior arm (Figs. 9.10A to C)
R	Roll the patient over on to all fours as it increases the pelvic diameters

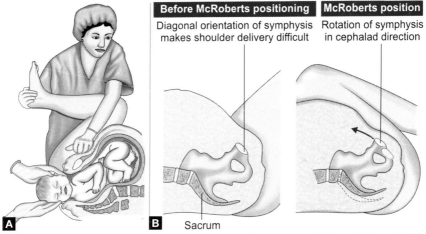

Figs. 9.5A and B: (A) McRoberts manoeuvre (exaggerated hyperflexion of the thighs upon the maternal abdomen) and application of suprapubic pressure; (B) McRoberts manoeuvre causes the pubic symphysis to rotate in cephalad direction and straightening of lumbosacral angle.

BMI, and foetal macrosomia. Therefore, the candidate's tutorial should be specially focused regarding the management of shoulder dystocia, a common complication associated with gestational diabetes.

• The candidate should conduct the teaching session objectively using the provided case scenario as an example. At the same time, they must be careful not to mention specific details related to the patient. They must simultaneously demonstrate their tutorial with reference to the props provided.

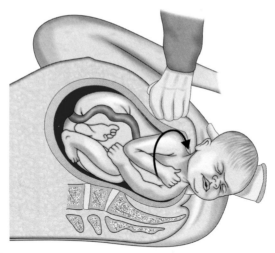

Fig. 9.6: Application of suprapubic pressure in the direction of foetal face.

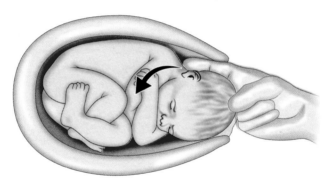

Fig. 9.7: Rubin II manoeuvre.

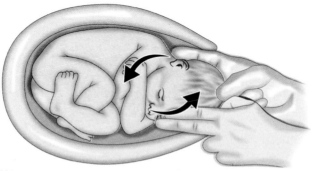

Fig. 9.8: Wood's screw manoeuvre: The hand is placed behind the posterior shoulder of the foetus. The shoulder is rotated progressively by 180° in a corkscrew manner so that the impacted anterior shoulder is released.

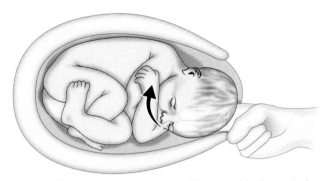

Fig. 9.9: Reverse Wood's screw manoeuvre: The shoulder is rotated progressively by 180° in a direction opposite to that described in the Wood' screw manoeuvre.

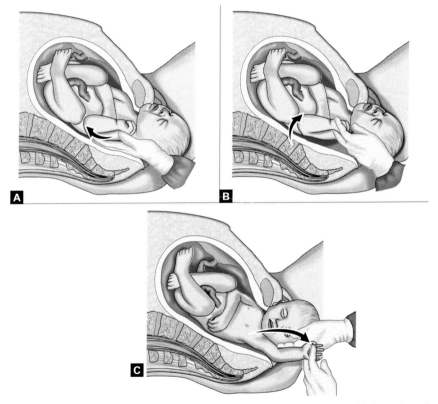

Figs. 9.10A to C: Delivery of posterior arm: (A) The clinician's hand is introduced into the vagina along the posterior shoulder. Keeping the arm flexed at the elbow, it is swept across the foetal chest; (B) The foetal hand is grasped and the arm is extended out along the side of the face; (C) The posterior arm and shoulder are delivered from the vagina.

Marking Scheme

0	1	2	3
Fail		Borderline	Pass

Recommendations

- An agreed guideline to be followed for training the labour staff regarding prompt management in cases of shoulder dystocia.
- Important to take up these concerns to a higher level.
- The Centre for Maternal and Child Enquiries (CMACE)/RCOG obesity guidelines must be followed while care of obese women.[14] RCOG guidelines must be followed while managing women with gestational diabetes.[15]
- Review the requirement for extra midwifery cover on the labour ward.
- Regular fire drills will help in ensuring that the expertise for management of shoulder dystocia is regularly updated.

Marking Scheme

0	1	2	3	4	5
Fail		Borderline		Pass	

Total score: /20

DISCUSSION

Issues

This type of OSCE station requires the candidate to think strategically about how they would be approaching the task. It is important that the candidate has a basic understanding about the principles and management of shoulder dystocia in order to pass this task because this is a skill which the candidate must have been using commonly in their routine clinical practice. Using the background of shoulder dystocia the candidate is expected to demonstrate more sophisticated skills, competencies, and attitudes, such as teaching skills, understanding of critical incidents, risk analysis, and participating in the clinical governance meetings.

Pitfalls

In tasks relating to adverse events, the candidate should take care to avoid assigning blame to any individual. This is a mechanism to prevent further similar adverse events. Putting blame on an individual can be considered as a potential mistake in this case. Another important flaw could be talking about management of shoulder dystocia with the examiner rather than discussing the technique for approaching the teaching session.

Variations

Various variations in these types of stations include a teaching session and risk analyses of any type of adverse invent which has been reported in obstetrics and gynaecology ward (Tables 9.1 and 9.2). Another variation in such kind of stations could be the occurrence of another complication such as Erb's paralysis due to overstretching of the baby's arms and shoulders while taking delivery in cases of shoulder dystocia.

OSCE STATION 5: AUDIT—THROMBOPROPHYLAXIS IN PATIENTS UNDERGOING GYNAECOLOGICAL SURGERY

Candidate's Instructions

An increase in the number of cases of venous thromboembolism (VTE) has been noted in patients who have had undergone gynaecological surgery in your ward. The nursing staff have looked at some of the cases and noticed that they have not all been administered mechanical thromboprophylaxis at the time of admission. Pharmacological thromboprophylaxis is also not correctly introduced in most patients.

You are asked to design an audit, for which you have 12 minutes (including 2 minutes of the reading time). You shall be awarded marks for the following tasks:

Candidate's tasks:

- Designing an audit
- Explaining the various steps of conducting an audit.

These tasks cover the domains as discussed next.

Core Clinical Skills Domains

Core clinical skills domains tested:

- Patient safety
- Communication with patients
- Communication with colleagues
- Information gathering
- Application of knowledge.

Module Tested

The modules tested in this station are Module 1 or 'Teaching' and Module 3 or 'Post-operative Care.'

EXAMINER'S INSTRUCTIONS AND STRUCTURED MARK SHEET

The examiner will mark the candidate on the basis of various tasks which are allotted to the candidate. The global score would be out of 40 marks, but the overall score for the station should be out of 20 marks by dividing the global score by 2. Each candidate task must be globally scored by the examiner.

Examiner's Instructions

Familiarise yourself with the candidate's instructions and the headings below. The candidate has 10 minutes to discuss his or her audit plan with you. Avoid prompting, and do not award half marks.

Designing an Audit

This would involve explaining the various steps of the audit process as discussed next.

Defining the Audit Topic

The use of venous thromboprophylaxis in women undergoing major gynaecological surgery.

Marking Scheme

0	1	2	3	4
Fail	Borderline		Pass	

Initial Needs Assessment

- Identifying the resources and assembling a multidisciplinary group
- Contacting the clinical risk and audit services
- Systematic review of evidence: literature, e.g. Medline, Cochrane, National Clinical Guidelines, and haematology input.
- Registering the audit project.

Marking Scheme

0	1	2	3	4	5	6
Fail		Borderline		Pass		

Defining a Standard

- Identifying the standards against which the audit will be compared. For this, the criteria for the current best practice need to be determined.
- In this case, this involves defining the proportion of compliance which constitutes good practice (100%).
- Defining the requirement for using mechanical VTE prophylaxis at the time of admission in all patients undergoing major gynaecological surgery.
- Mechanical VTE prophylaxis could include thigh or knee length anti-embolism stockings, foot impulse devices or intermittent pneumatic compression devices.
- May need to define which pharmacological anticoagulant strategy should be used in patients with low risk of bleeding depending on haematology advice:

- Need to choose between low molecular weight heparin or unfractionated heparin
- Pharmacological thromboprophylaxis must be continued until the patient no longer has significantly reduced mobility (generally 5–7 days).

Marking Scheme

0	1	2	3	4	5	6
Fail		Borderline		Pass		

Data Collection and Analysis

- The methodology for data collection as well as who is going to collect the data is to be decided.
- Either the sample size (number of cases for the audit) or the audit timelines need to be defined.
- Needs to decide whether to conduct a retrospective or prospective audit.
- Defining the audit sample (in this case, all patients undergoing major gynaecological surgery).
- Consider risk factors for the development of VTE (e.g. surgery for gynaecological malignancy; BMI >30 kg/m^2; history of VTE in the family; using hormonal replacement therapy or oral contraceptives; varicose veins; prolonged immobilisation, etc.)
- Designing a pro forma for collection of valid and reliable data.
- Entering the collected data onto a spreadsheet.
- Appropriate analysis and interpretation of the collected data.

Marking Scheme

0	1	2	3	4	5	6
Fail		Borderline		Pass		

Presenting Recommendations and Implementing Changes to Improve Care

- Providing recommendations to individuals and units involved in the care of these patients.
- Identifying areas, where changes need to be implemented (e.g. individuals, organisational changes, mechanical thromboprophylaxis to be initiated in all patients at the time of admission; pharmacological thromboprophylaxis to be initiated in patients who have a low risk of major bleeding, taking into account individual patient factors based on the clinical judgement).[16]
- Identify sources of resistance to change and anticipate potential problems, adopting a proactive approach to solve them.
- Reviewing medical practice as discussed above and using appropriate forums for the dissemination of recommendations.

- Disseminating changes and new standards via e-mail, newsletters, noticeboard bulletin, flyers, and grand round-type meeting.
- Defining a time period for the implementation of these changes.

Marking Scheme

0	1	2	3	4	5	6
Fail		Borderline		Pass		

Re-audit

- Defining a suitable timeline for re-audit, usually within 12 months of changes.
- Re-audit results would need to be re-evaluated to see if more changes are necessary to further improve the clinical outcome.

Marking Scheme

0	1	2	3	4	5	6
Fail		Borderline		Pass		

Global Score

This is based on the examiner's overall assessment of the candidate.

0	1	2	3	4	5	6
Poor	Below average	Borderline		Good	Excellent	

Total score: /40 = score/2 =/20

DISCUSSION

Issues

In such kind of stations, it is important for the candidate to read the task carefully and realise that they need to mainly design an audit in this case. The best strategy to answer such types of question is to break the answer into small fragments by describing each individual step involved in the audit process. The examiner may have been asked to individually score each step and then to give a global score based on the overall performance of the candidate. Therefore, clear description of each individual step is extremely important in this case.

In this station, while devising a pro forma for using venous thrombo-prophylaxis in women undergoing major gynaecological surgery, the candidate's search must focus on the current incidence of VTE; the groups at high risk for developing VTE; and the current best practice for prevention of VTE in patients undergoing major gynaecological surgery. Once the pro forma has been designed, it must be distributed amongst various stake holders such as general practitioners, theatre and ward nurses, consultant surgeons, etc. The recommendations to be instituted in the unit are then decided following a discussion between various stakeholders. These are then implemented, following which the data related to outcome needs to be analysed. This helps in evaluating if a particular protocol is demonstrating a benefit to the unit or not.

Pitfalls

Describing the various steps of audit all together, without clearly describing each step in details, is likely to result in failure. The candidate must carefully read the question to understand what they are really required to do.

Variations

Designing an audit in a particular OSCE station could be related to any of the condition which is not being properly managed in the department. However, the process of designing an audit more or less remains the same. Audit may also be required for issues holding high priority for one's department/trust or hospital, e.g. areas with a high volume of work load or those having an increased rate of mortality and morbidity. The candidate must keep in mind various such issues which could serve as a potential topic for an audit.

REFERENCES

1. Scally G, Donaldson LJ. Clinical governance and the drive for quality improvement in the new NHS in England. BMJ. 1998;317(7150):61-5.
2. Department of Health. A First Class Service: Quality in the New NHS. HMSO: London; 1998.
3. Starey N. (2001). What is clinical governance? Evidence-based medicine, Hayward Medical Communications. [online] Available from goo.gl/qpySYU [Accessed December 2017].
4. NHS litigation Authority. Ten years of maternity claims: An analysis of NHS litigation authority data. London: NHSLA; 2012.
5. Royal College of Obstetricians and Gynaecologists. Improving patient safety: risk management for maternity and gynaecology. Clinical Governance Advice No. 2. London: RCOG; 2009.
6. National Patient Safety Agency. (2010). Root cause analysis: fishbone template. [online] Available from http://www. nrls.npsa.nhs.uk/resources/?entryid45=75605 [Accessed October 2017].
7. National Institute for Health and Clinical Excellence. Principles for Best Practice in Clinical Audit. 2002. [online] Available from http://www.nice.org.uk/media/796/23/BestPracticeClinicalAudit.pdf [Accessed October 2017].
8. NHS Clinical Governance Support Group. A Practical Handbook for Clinical Audit (2005). [online] Available from www.dvh.nhs.uk/EasySiteWeb/GatewayLink.aspx?alId=107269 [Accessed October 2017].
9. Smith R. Audit and research. BMJ. 1992;305:905-6.
10. Royal College of Obstetricians and Gynaecologists. The Investigation and Management of the Small–for–Gestational–Age Fetus. Green-top Guideline No. 31. London: RCOG; 2014.
11. Alberry M, Soothill P. Management of fetal growth restriction. Arch Dis Child Fetal Neonatal Ed. 2007;92(1):F62-F67.

12. Leung TY, Stuart O, Sahota DS, et al. Head-to-body delivery interval and risk of fetal acidosis and hypoxic ischaemic encephalopathy in shoulder dystocia: a retrospective review. BJOG. 2011;118(4):474-9.
13. Royal College of Obstetricians and Gynaecologists. Shoulder Dystocia. Green–top Guideline No. 42, 2nd edition. London: RCOG; 2012.
14. Royal College of Obstetricians and gynaecologists and Centre for Maternal and Child Enquiries (CMACE). CMACE/RCOG Joint Guidelines for management of women with obesity in pregnancy. London: RCOG; 2010.
15. Royal College of Obstetricians and gynaecologists. Diagnosis and Treatment of Gestational Diabetes. Scientific Impact Paper No. 23. London: RCOG; 2011.
16. National Institute of clinical Excellence. (2010). Venous thromboembolism: reducing the risk for patients in hospital. Clinical guideline [CG92]. Updated 2015. London: NICE.

Index

Page numbers followed by *f* refer to figure, *fc* refers to flow chart and *t* refers to table.